"*Enlightening…. All too often, medical professionals focus on facts and figures… but may lose sight of the patient in front of us. Abbe's book helps us remember this and guides us through an experience that is unique for each individual. I highly recommend this book for patients and families undergoing the sometimes confusing, often fearful, and yes, at times even joyful, process of cancer care.*"

- **Dr. Bruce Mathey, North Puget Cancer Center, Peace Health United General Medical Center.**

"*Cocoon of Cancer is a poetic, poignant, and scientifically accurate memoir. Abbe's Caregiver's Tips add insights to those who will identify with similar thoughts and feelings.*"

- **Dr. Fred Appelbaum, Executive Vice President, Fred Hutchinson Cancer Research Center Executive Director & President, Seattle Cancer Care Alliance.**

"*One cannot help but fully enter [the authors'] world as life around them at home and in the hospital evolves. Similar to Helene Hanff's post World War II book,* **84 Charing Cross Rd,** *today's* **COCOON OF CANCER** *evokes the same intimacy of interchange, recording the candid tenderness and fears that surface for Abbe and Jim… This book will be a source of comfort, support, and information to couples entering the foreign world of high-tech cancer care while preserving their sense of family.*"

~ **Dr. Stewart B Fleishman, Founding Director, Cancer Supportive Services, Continuum Cancer Centers of New York, part of Mt. Sinai Health System; Author,** *Learn to Live Through Cancer: What You Need to Know and Do.*

Other books by Abbe Rolnick:

River of Angels (2010)   •   *Color of Lies* (2013)

Abbe Rolnick
with Jim Wiggins

**Cocoon of Cancer:
An Invitation To Love Deeply**

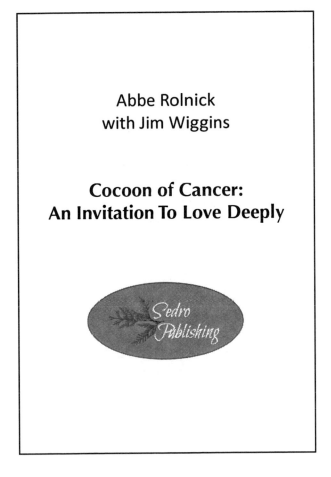

Cocoon of Cancer: An Invitation To Love Deeply / Abbe Rolnick with Jim Wiggins, First edition.

Sedro Publishing,
21993 Grip Road,
Sedro Woolley, WA 98284
www.sedropublishing.com.

Library of Congress Control Number: 2015911229

ISBN 978-0-9845119-3-8 (trade book)
ISBN 978-0-9845119-4-5 (electronic book)

Cover design and prepress by Karen Parker (www.karenparkerdesigns.com).

Editorial Assistance: Sara Stamey (www.sarastamey.com).

Illustrations by Barbara Defreytas (see more of her illustrations @ www.sedropublishing.com.)

Cocoon of Cancer: An Invitation to Love Deeply
Abbe Rolnick with Jim Wiggins

Awe has to do with grace: The ability to see, feel, and act with broad appreciation. If this is faith, then faith is synonymous with god. Would Awe have form and rules?

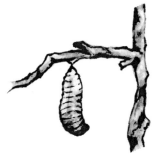

Finite ends, but infinity still exists. So my friend, lover, and infinite man, another day in Paradise begins.

What we know keeps us sane, until time opens and reveals more nuggets of knowledge.

What we know keeps us humble, until time opens the door.

What we know keeps us on the path, until we walk through.

I wish I could speak for all those with cancer, all those in pain. I speak for myself and hope others can benefit.

- Abbe Rolnick

Contents

Acknowledgments

I thank those who have helped Jim and me through our journey with cancer. To Jim's siblings Gracie, Richard, Larry, Steve, and Johnny, who cared for him with words of encouragement, time, and stem cells. Richard, you endured so many procedures to assure Jim would have your stem cells and another chance to live. Johnny, you sat with Jim and kept his spirits up. To my mother Selma, who held on tight with a brightness and will. My sister Harriet lent her ear, and my three children Mara, Will, and Elly kept me grounded with visits, food, and laughter.

Janet and Garth, we hope to pay forward as you two have with the lending of your condo to us for seven months.

Karla, you kept Jim's business going. Thank you for your help.

Cheryll and Gary, your homemade beef, chicken, and vegetable broths nourished both of us with the nutrients of love. Your homemade fruit popsicles sweetened our dark days.

Calls and cards from friends, family, colleagues, and strangers brightened our days. Special thanks to Wendy, who searched for housing and called with laughter. Jan, you traveled with me on book talks, drove when my fear took over, and shared my moods. Shirley, your strength held us together. Teri, you have been my rock throughout my entire life. You keep me sane.

The staff at North Puget Cancer Center (Peace Health United General), along with Dr. Bruce Mathey's insightful care, set us on the healing path. Seattle Cancer Care Alliance gave us all their expertise and individual care. A special thanks to Dr. William Bensinger and Dr. Frederick Appelbaum for their diligence in searching for cancer cures. The Violet and Red Team of nurses, physician assistants, doctors, and schedulers, you all are family. More thanks, hugs, and the proverbial "hang in there."

And to my editor Sara Stamey, publicist Alice Acheson, and illustrator Barbara Defreytas, your talents helped give form to our words.

Caregiver Tips, Questions I Still Ponder, and *Questions the Reader Should Ponder* are included at the close of this manuscript. These are meant for all caregivers, the inquisitive, cancer survivors, and readers who would like to open discussions among themselves or with loved ones.

∞

Prologue

This is what we knew before we knew my husband had cancer: In October of 2013, Jim slipped on the last rung of a ladder while watering in the greenhouse that held his precious orchids. Jim considered the soreness that followed a nuisance. Two days out on his annual elk hunt, he returned home early with pain so severe that his legs crumpled. He could not bend or twist. X-rays and a doctor's diagnosis stated he had osteopenia, one collapsed vertebrae, and a few fractures. The doctor's advice was to rest for a month and add calcium and vitamin D to his diet. Simple.

Strong, healthy, and stubborn, Jim never complained. He rested. He hurt. He knew he would heal, he always had. We left on a planned trip to Africa in December. Three weeks of what the safari guides call the African massage—rutted roads—kept Jim in pain. He photographed the lions, hippos, rhinos, and giraffes, until all he could manage was to sit and watch the magnificent birds of the Serengeti.

Home again, Jim held on to the belief he would heal. Somehow he felt guilty of exacerbating the pain through our African adventure. He waited until finally the pain was too much, and three months later he returned for more X-rays. I got the call, the one every person dreads. "Abbe, can you come home? I have cancer."

∞

∞

False Healing
February 19, 2014

In the oncologist office as they perform a bone marrow biopsy on Jim. I sit on the sidelines, avoiding seeing the procedure to keep from fainting.

I love Jim Wiggins
I love Jim Wiggins
I love Jim Wiggins
I love Jim Wiggins
I don't want him to die. I want to live with him forever and be the best wife, friend, and lover. I want my life to be entwined with his blue eyes, his soft hands, his exuberance with nature, his passion. I love the way he loves me.
I will not be selfish.
I will give all that I can.
I will write and touch others' hearts for him.
I am here to give more love.
I am a conduit of joy.
I will not suffer. I will enjoy and give Jim all my humor and my crazy bits of wisdom. I will keep our connection. I might be scared, but fear isn't anything to be ashamed of. Fear makes me grow, if not taller, then deeper. My heart expands with the "L" words: Love, Like, Listen, Luck, and Laughter.

I place a pen between my lips so I won't offer my thoughts when Jim is listening or talking to the doctor. I want to scream my thoughts...but I smile, pretending I can find the humor, kindness, and grace. I want no regrets.

∞

I focus on keeping the calm as the storm swirls. And to remember best intentions, not an easy task, to keep Jim comfortable.

Lots of kissing...

Dinner at the Wiggins/ Rolnick Home on February 19, 2014

Haiku from Jim

Home from our doc talk.
Dinner, digesting the day
Can't speak, overwhelmed.

John calls, how are we?
Two thoughts are all I can say,
Eating, have cancer.

Email from Jim,
February 20, 2014

Hello all, more of the story:

In October I "broke" my back but did not realize it. Went hunting, and my back hurt so bad I had to leave early. Returned home and went to the doctor in early November and had an x-ray done. The doctor said I had a compression fracture in my 4th lumbar, and osteopenia. So he put me on some vitamins and drugs. Hobbled through November and then went to Africa, where the rough roads did not help the back pain. After returning home I waited a few weeks to see a doctor and finally saw one in early February.

This is where the story changes. All this time I thought I was on the mend, but when I had an MRI done the doctor said I had more cracks in my vertebrae, and some of the vertebrae were reduced in size, in other words the damn things were disappearing. I then had a blood test (this all happened yesterday), which showed a high level of protein cells, and I was anemic. With this information, the doctor now believes I have Multiple Myeloma. He then took a bone marrow sample from my hip, and the results from that test will be available tomorrow. I have an appointment with the doc to go over all the results, which will confirm if I do indeed have MM. I do suspect I have MM, and if so, I will start on chemotherapy soon. Not sure what other therapies he'll prescribe, but will find out tomorrow. I'll let you know what I find out. Abbe and I have a lot of talking to do to make sure our lives are in order for what is coming at us.

M & M no longer evokes the image of candy, but multiple myeloma.

∞

Email from Janet,
February 20, 2014

Jim and Abbe,

I am so sorry to hear about the Multiple Myeloma diagnosis. Garth and I will keep you in our prayers for the biopsy to be negative for the MM. I am so glad you have each other for support and that you are such a positive, optimistic couple. And don't forget all the rest of your family and friends who love you and are pulling for you, too. There will be lots of prayers being said and loads of great Karma filling the atmosphere on your behalf.

Love and Peace,
Janet and Garth

Email from Abbe to Frances,
February 22, 2014

Life has its twists and turns. This bend of the road is a sharp one—especially with the speed. Jim's fractured back turned out to be not a fracture caused by natural causes. While we thought he was healing, the plasma cells in the bone marrow multiplied too quickly and overtook his normal blood cells. This caused anemia and leakage of an acid that is eating away at his spine and other bones. They call this multiple myeloma. He is in Stage Three—the most advanced for this type of cancer. We start chemo on Monday, and if we can get the readings down from 80% to 10%, Jim will have a stem cell transplant, where they harvest his stem cells, and after radiation and more chemotherapy the harvested cells are replaced inside Jim. All this takes place at Fred Hutchinson Cancer Care Center in Seattle. That would happen, if we are lucky, in about three months. Jim is Jim, not complaining, looking at this as a scientist.

We will carry on our lives as close to the normal as possible. However, Jim is in pain, tires easily, and is very vulnerable to catching germs. So we invite our friends to call and pop in when we are home. I'll be here most of the time (home) with short jaunts to Robeks to make sure all is well with the business.

We are lucky that our home, life, love, family, and friends are so wonderful.

Best always,
Abbe

∞

Healing

I believe in the warmth between the pains.
I believe that I can kiss the air and the love moves with
it.
I believe that if I can see your eye, I see your heart.
I believe healing comes with laughter.
So...I will curl with you, find your funny bones.
Kiss the air and warm your heart.
Here is to you feeling better.

Email from Abbe to Adrian,
February 25, 2014

Adrian,

I so appreciate your kind thoughts and wishes. The
cancer journey is one no one chooses.

Jim's question isn't why me, but why me now? I am
taking each step in sync with Jim's. He is my loving
companion, special in all ways. Neither of us has a
choice. He worries about the pain he inflicts on his
friends and family. You are correct, so many people are
here to support us.

Our goal is to reduce Jim's plasma cells down from 80%
to the 10% required for the stem cell transplant.

The first chemotherapy appointment yesterday was
tough. A blizzard of heavy snow knocked out power

lines, our generator failed, and I found myself outside with a small hand saw, cutting down limbs to get us out of our driveway. Hands frozen, after two sets of twenty-minute intervals, I answered my daughter's call to my cell phone. Hearing the desperation in my voice, she called Jim's brother who lives in town, a thirty-minute drive from our home.

Jim had no idea of Elly's rescue call. Later I explained to Jim that it was a job for a chainsaw, and I don't do chainsaw. I had him laughing, which broke the ice, pun intended.

So my friend Adrian, I thank you for all that you give from afar, for being a cancer model who understands.

Best always,
Abbe

Awaiting Sweet Nectar

Jim has embarked on an unsolicited journey. A traveler, scientist, and adventurer, he sees the world with eyes of wonder and discovery. Jim is one of the chosen few given the opportunity to be humbled in the wake of living. His new journey takes us both into territory that has dubious directions and a cloudy beginning. Unlike our trips to Sri Lanka, Kenya, Puerto Rico, or along the Columbia River, the cancer journey embodies the abstract concept of living with the end in sight.

Each day brings miracles to our window. We watch the seasons change with the presence of birds—Stellar Jays forever present, and now with the buds bursting on our trees, the hummingbirds return seeking sweetened water until flowers blossom. Jim walks slowly, filling feeders with sunflower seeds, suet, and peanuts. He sits in his big brown chair by the living room window, delighted with the flit-flight of old friends and the scurried activity of squirrels and rabbits.

Protocol takes us to our local cancer center—radiation, chemotherapy, blood draws, doctor visits. Now that we're into our eighth week, the receptionists, nurses, lab technicians, doctors, and even the cleaning staff know us by first names. Jim, with his corny sense of humor, ribs the red-headed lab technician who draws his blood: "I'll be seeing you for the next thirty years. Take care of yourself." And if he is lucky, that will be the truth. For Jim's cancer isn't curable, and the red-haired lady will turn gray but still greet him with the same, "Here comes Jim Wiggins. I've got you."

∞

Blood, the lifeline for all living creatures, passes through Jim with too many plasma cells. We watch weekly as the chemo attacks the M-proteins, myeloma. Questions upon questions multiply, as Jim puts together the puzzle of mutations and the effects of too much cloning. Cause and effect, consequences, experiments, these words belong to science, and Jim relies on new technology to pave his chances of thriving past two and on to ten years.

Even on our off weeks, when Jim's body rests from chemo or radiation, I drive us to the cancer center, ten minutes from our home in the Skagit Valley to what becomes a second home. It is luck that sends us to the oldest cancer treatment center north of Seattle. Tests take time, give answers to unasked questions. There is a sense of comfort between patients. I console the newlywed lady, wracked with grief and anguish at her husband's diagnosis. "What do I do with my anger?"

She wants me to fix a problem as if there is an answer. I hug the stranger and feel her tears on my face. "Dig a big hole with a large, heavy shovel. Then drop every ounce of anger into the pit. Find a beautiful plant to place within the hole, cover the roots, and watch it grow." Her husband mouths "thank-you" as he heads off to radiation.

On our way to a bone-marrow biopsy, we pass Larry, a throat cancer patient, who befriended Jim on the first day of chemotherapy. In a room filled with fellow adventurers, each with their formulated chemical cocktails, Larry had noticed Jim's discomfort as he struggled in the overstuffed chair. Although he couldn't speak, Larry motioned to Jim to pull the lever on the side, to ease the legs up. Small gestures have huge significance. Jim and I both note that Larry feels poorly, but even though his cancer has affected his face, Larry's eyes hold us. We watch as he heads to radiation, a sign that his cancer has taken another detour.

Time slows to a standstill, absorbing the needs of all around us. Everyone, staff and patients, develops a choreographed dance based on need and urgency. Rooms fill up, and they shift Jim into a room across the way, an official operating room in the hospital. Our nurse follows, and soon Dr. Bruce Mathey makes his entrance. He remembers all our conversations and engages Jim in the science of probing. More aware of the pain of the procedure the second time around, Jim talks less. The doctor fills the void with a prediction. "I believe the results will show the plasma cells have been reduced from 80% to 15%." Jim and I hope for the same.

Soon Jim will graduate from our local cancer center to the renowned Seattle Cancer Care Alliance. As the hummingbirds wait for the flower blossoms, Jim waits for the M-proteins and plasma cells to disappear. His sweet nectar will come from stem cell transplants, one from his own and one from a matching donor. As the physical pain subsides, his eyes tear up. He isn't afraid of dying. He loves his life and feels only the immense weight of gratitude and the sadness of causing emotional pain for others. I am a companion on this journey, blessed with the grace to be open to uncertainty.

Email from Mike to Abbe,
February 26, 2014

Abbe,

I wanted to check in after receiving your email forwarded by Sue. I am very sorry to hear the news about Jim and promise as you requested in your email to love, laugh, learn, and live life fully both personally and with others in support of both your and Jim's journey.

Along the way please feel free to reach for me for anything that you two might need. I don't care if you decide you want an apple at two in the morning or need a jacket placed over a puddle, I am here for you both. I have quite a tool box full of resources that can figure out a way to get you whatever might make things easier or more comfortable. Please don't ever hesitate to call, text, fax, or email. I have my cell with me 24/7.

In the meantime, I will keep you both in my thoughts and prayers as well as send positive energy your way.

Love to you my friend,
Mike

Email from Abbe to Frances,
March 5, 2014

Another hard day. Jim's pain is so evident that the nurses and doctors are concerned. This was our second day of radiation as we continue the twice weekly chemo treatments. We are at the clinic every day for

∞

radiation, ten total. We will have the official in-person consult at the SCCA soon, but no date yet. My hope is to get ahead of the cancer, as it is running out of control. Jim looks at me with his puppy dog eyes, blue oceans, saying so much. Braving the moment.

**Email from Frances in response,
March 5, 2014**

Abbe,
This is breaking my heart. And yours too, I'm sure. I share your hope that these difficult treatments will fight back the cancer and give Jim a chance of feeling better and living longer. My love to both of you.

**Email from Abbe,
March 5, 2014**

Jim is sleeping, and he doesn't want to get up. My heart hasn't hurt this much ever. Elly is coming to cook us a dinner, but I know Jim will pass on it. I hope he will eat later, as all the medicines require food. Our consult for the SCCA is now set for March 19th, after radiation, and between chemo sessions.
Not much else. I can't concentrate.

- Me

**Email from Harriet,
March 5, 2014**

Dear Abbe,

I have thought about you so many times today, but did not call as I know you need some time and space from the well-meaning callers. I can't begin to imagine how overwhelmed you are feeling with it all. But I have no doubt that your indomitable spirit, natural optimism, deep abiding love, and the support of all of those who love you and Jim will see you through things. I know you know I am here for you and Jim. My life and work are completely consuming, but I can change what I am doing and extricate myself from it all to help you. I love you, plain and simple. There is little I would not do for you.

So on that note, my dear sister, please call when you can. I am thinking about you and sending all my love and most positive of thoughts and prayers.

**Email from Abbe to Harriet,
March 6, 2014**

Dearest Harriet,

Yesterday afternoon and evening were the hardest yet. I came home from work to a very pained Jim. He is no longer driving. At the radiation appointment, our nurse noticed Jim's stiffness and pain and immediately called the doctor to get him another medicine. They made him understand that his body can't go with the ups and downs of pain and that he shouldn't wait for some sign to take his painkiller. The body reacts negatively to the dip.

He fell asleep in the car while I ran errands, and when he took off his clothes to let me apply oils for his radiated body, he just slept. I gave him a smoothie so he could take more medication for the night.

Elly came and cooked. The two of us ate quietly. If she hadn't come, I would have skipped eating, as I was drained. She left and I went to bed.

I held Jim's hand most of the night. This morning he asked about all the phone calls (business, employees, doctors, and friends). I took messages for all that I could, except when the SCCA called, and I had to get his permission for them to talk with me. We go down on March 19th, an 8:00 AM consult for four hours. John and Jan will drive us, as we have to leave here early and the day will be long. I don't know how much Jim will be able to walk. I'm going to ask for a handicap parking pass, and we'll see if he will need a wheelchair. I'm hoping that after next week's radiation and a break in the chemo, he'll regain some energy.

Seeing Jim in such pain is the hard part. He doesn't want to think about anything but relief. I want to give him this. I'll massage him later this morning. I won't go into work today, as we have radiation, chemo, and another doctor consult. Maybe I'll run in for a couple of hours on Friday. Thanks for your note, love, and desire to help.

∞

Email from Jim to friend Andy,
March 6, 2014

Good to hear from you.

Here's a quick rundown from a layman's perspective. I have multiple myeloma. The trigger is a mutant gene (no kidding). The gene is P-53 on my 17th chromosome. Said gene inhibits cell growth, and although I am not sure, I believe it specifically deals with blood cells. My P-53 gene mutated and does not inhibit the plasma cell growth anymore. In my case, my plasma cells are cloning themselves. So I am in a cloning war with a mutant gene. (I'm told that the P-53 gene behaves differently in other cancers.)

The problem is the plasma cells are crowding out the rest of the cells in my blood, hindering my other blood cells (white cells and red cells) from doing their job. Somewhere along the line the plasma clones are affecting the calcium in my body and accumulating in specific places such as my spine. Thus my spine is getting weaker and hurts like hell.

The chemo affects all fast-growing cells, and the radiation is targeting the specific areas where my bone density is decreasing. I mentioned my spine, but also my upper left arm and my left hip have reduced bone density.

I go to Seattle in two weeks to have a meeting with the Seattle Cancer Care Alliance to discuss a stem cell transplant.

Note from Abbe to Jim,
March 2014

I hear your voice explain the significance of the garden aesthetics. I don't presume to know what the definition includes in your mind. But as I look out and see the newly planted rows of cabbage and lettuce, see the posts of future dahlias, spot the rising posts of sweet peas, and visualize the pots of tomatoes, I know that nature will take over and keep the cycle of green leaves, buds, flowers, and fruit. Even if the weeds come and we are absent, the aesthetics exist. We don't have to see it to feel the vibrant cycles, the lushness of a garden's seasons. The garden doesn't belong to us alone; the privilege is shared among the birds and animals. The bounty lies with the process: planting, watering, harvesting, and the beauty of stages. My thoughts probe your word, aesthetics.

Vision:
Seeing isn't believing.

Green fills the window. Yellow sun shines through dark clouds. Almost blinded, my eyes focus on the pale green dogwood tree whose branches rise high to peek above the window sill. Vanilla flowers open skyward, unnoticed from the ground. For some reason this makes me smile, as if the dogwood tree has a secret that only I can see. And these—the beauty, the flowers—exist even if no one can see them.

Jim's cancer is invisible. I can't see his plasma cells overproducing, eating away at his bones. All I see is a shorter Jim, whose body has shrunk three inches in response. His deep blue eyes twinkle less, drier as a result of the chemo cocktail, but if it is early in the day and his energy is with him, the sparkle comes through with a morning smile. I crave kisses and seek his lips often. I know that our passion lies in wait. Memories fill my heart as I refocus my perception of what our lives entail.

There are moments when I forget that cancer inhabits our world. Jim says he too forgets, but for him the cancer sits firmly on his left shoulder, whispering into his ear the moment he lets his guard down. I don't suffer the fatigue, the effects of steroids changing my shape, or the dryness, hunger, discomforts. Yet I'm on alert, as if each of my cells battles the invisible plasma cells within Jim.

Progress means that Jim will get sicker before he improves. Of his four brothers, hopefully one is a match for a stem cell transplant. As a donor, he will be Jim's path to a future. The closer the match, the less chance of rejection. Rejection, a denial of self. First, Jim will have his own stem cells harvested to replenish his bone marrow. He'll ingest another, more potent chemo cocktail that will attack his immune system. Hopefully he won't reject himself, and when the second round of transplant follows he'll remain strong, while his brother's stem cells attack the remaining myeloma. The battle seems so violent. I want to call a truce to explain the rules of engagement. "Stem cells, attack only the myeloma, shake hands with all the other cells. Keep my Jim safe."

Jim's secret strength is invisible from the outside, like the upside-down dogwood flowers. I see him best with my eyes closed, as I spoon in bed. We hold hands in the dark. The intimacy of a disease, the sharing of hearts, reaches way beyond the sky. I have no idea of where the cancer will take us, but we continue opening our petals. This is my secret. I value Jim's inner strength even as he is weakened. I see green and yellow, hope and warmth. We don't talk about the dark hole of what ifs. I only ask for more kisses. I'm greedy, but I too hear the cancer whispering in my ear. And when this happens, I keep my eyes sealed, roll over, and let the dreams and visions of beauty encircle us.

Email from Abbe to writing mentor Mary, March 6, 2014

It is only two weeks into our journey. I'm exhausted. Jim is struggling. Our race is a hard one. The cancer is more aggressive than we'd expected, and the race between treatments and getting ahead of the course takes a toll. I thought you'd appreciate this poem.

Erasing

I no longer know the days.
Just the rhythm of chemo,
radiation, pills swallowed.

Nurses, patients, become
friends of necessity
now more comfortable

than the well-meaning
loves who ache with
phantom pain.

Days dissolve years.
Time travel accelerated
erasing futures.

Hope lies within
hands entwined
bedside buddies

Whose passion dreams
connect fibers
New DNA.

∞

Email from Jim to Cheryll,
March 8, 2014

Yes, I did begin radiation treatment on Tuesday. It continues for another six days, ten total. I don't really feel the effects, no skin burn yet and don't expect any, can't really tell what it is doing inside of me. They are targeting my spine, upper left arm, and left hip because those locations are where the plasma cells are concentrating and reducing my bone density. The radiation should stop the loss of bone.

John and Jan will be driving us to the SCCA. We'll be going over all the details of the bone marrow transplant (also called stem and T cell transplant) with them. I can tell you more after that appointment. From what I read, it is a rigorous procedure, but I do not know how long that part of the journey will last. Too many questions to answer right now, and it also depends on the effectiveness of my current chemo and radiation treatments.

Email from Abbe to Frances,
March, 2014

Our journey meanders with physical pain, tiredness, and the emotional roller-coaster that accompanies these bodily changes. Add to this the not-knowing. It is both peaceful and fraught with danger.

Jim is resting after his radiation. His pain level is very high, and we will get a new medication tomorrow after a doctor's consult and another radiation treatment. This is the off-week for his chemo shot. He has three more chemo pills that are very toxic, and then we start again on Monday.

Our next adventure, the one to SCCA, is perhaps the scariest. I'll be the caregiver, which means I take on the role of nurse, learning to administer intravenous medicine through the eventual port. We have no idea of when or how long we will be gone. Stay tuned for the news.

Jim is fascinated by the idea that he is fighting a war with a cloning plasma cell and a mutant P-53 gene (an inhibitor that stopped inhibiting).

Mara and AJ had dinner with us on Saturday night, and when Mara went to a baby shower on Sunday, AJ worked in the yard. I did, too, pruning all the sad-looking ferns. Jim's brother Richard and kids came to visit.

Not much else.

- Abbe

Email from Jim to Abbe at work, March, 2014

Abbe,
I have more energy today or
maybe I don't hurt as much, or
maybe emotionally, I am becoming more optimistic
(back to my old self)?
I believe it is all three.

The new pain relief pills cut the major pain but still
keep me aware of my body.
It remains an enigma as to how poorly one can feel yet
feel good.
Also, the emotions of...
Why now?
What is really going on?
What else ails me?
Where did it come from?
What is the process of working with cancer?
And finally, life is good and I shall prevail
Together

- Jim

Email reply from Abbe to Jim,
March, 2014

You are an amazing man-boy
complex and innocent
strong and vulnerable
optimism with relief
Allow cycles to
spring alive
Questions
Answers
More questions
Together possibilities

- Me

Email from Abbe to friends and family, March, 2014

We two are blessed that so many small acts make us happy. I work when I can get to Robeks, usually leaving early for a swim and putting in four hours at the café. Family and friends have helped us with food, digging me out of the snow, and general yard work. My kids rally with support, and Jim's large family helps by just being there for him. After our consult in Seattle next week, we'll have to find a place to live for months (four to seven). We can only be fifteen minutes away from SCCA for all the procedures.

This morning the rains have ceased, and I see an opportunity to walk to our mailbox for the Sunday paper. I'll work in our greenhouse for a short while, and if I can, write the next chapter of my new novel, *Founding Stones.*

Jim and I hold hands with more love than seems possible. Something about the curve of our hands, the warmth, and the edge of worn muscles gives us the texture that sustains our hearts. We are blessed that our windows open out to nature, and we see all the birds bringing in new life and the green of spring. We watch, read, listen, and are content.

This journey is not our choice, but one we must take. Jim does not like it that his pain causes pain for others. He is a wise scientist, a loving man, and when he gets the opportunity, he has a sense of humor that keeps me going.

Mara, my oldest, is four months pregnant. She is funnier

∞

than funny with all her issues. She makes me smile. We look forward to a baby. Elly pops in weekly with food and fun. Will comes in with male energy, ready to chop wood and remove physical pressures.

With that, I'll end this note. The rains have returned. Breakfast is calling, and the house, cozy with a fire in the woodstove, welcomes a leisured Sunday.

Much love,
Abbe

Still at home, a note from Abbe to Jim, March 2014

You talk about a bucket list, and there is so much for us to do. Let's get our list together, and when we are on the other side of the cancer adventure, we'll take the time. Thanks for gardening, thanks for organizing the recycling shelves. Thanks for falling asleep in the "V" of my lap.

Note from Abbe to Jim, March 15, 2014

I'm struck by color. Greens, soft, dark, and light-filled with yellow and blue and outrageous red flowers. Rhododendrons' pompous blooms and the quiet vanilla white of the false lily of the valley, elegant against the tall green stems. Brown turns to fluffy green fiddle fronds as the ferns unravel. Crab apple trees surprise us with pink/red flowers contrasting with the cherry blossoms a hue lighter. The yellow daffodils, long gone, ushered in the spring, and now a lush emerald-green carpet surrounds the gardens. Even in the morning, muted colors wait for the dark sky to lift. Sunshine on a dreary day colors our life.

**Email from Abbe to Teri,
March 19, 2014**

The sun just decided to climb out from behind the rain clouds. I'll take that as a showing from the universe that Jim's journey is on the fast track and that all will progress in a rainbow arc, with health and thriving as a culminating goal.

We had our consult at the SCCA today. Our doctor didn't mince words—told us what we suspected: Jim's multiple myeloma is on the fast track. We must beat the race with aggressive chemo and then have two stem cell transplants. One from his own stem cells and then another almost immediately from a donor. Because he has the mutant P-53 gene, an inhibitor that has been deleted, his own stem cells can't totally stop the myeloma. Only with another source can he kill off all of them. They call the P-53 a prognostic determiner. Without the second transplant from a donor, he has about two to three years of life expectancy. The second stem cell transplant has its risks. Lots of complications due to rejection, infection, and some really big names, but if Jim responds well, we have given him perhaps another nine years. Now we have to see if his siblings are a match. If not, we may or may not have a second stem cell transplant as an option. The big unknown.

Most likely we will proceed to Seattle in June or July

for 145 days, five months or more. This is more than I bargained for. Yes, support I can give, but who knew that I'd be a city girl, acting as a caregiver for my wonderful Jim. I keep finding blessings: If our insurance gives prior approval, we won't have to pay $1 million.

I will be looking for spotters, those who can replace me and still keep Jim comfortable, when I have to return to Bellingham. He won't be able to be alone. I'm sure it will work out with my kids, Jim's family, and friends. We'll plant flowers in our garden instead of vegetables. Mowing and watering will keep our sanctuary ready for our return. I'll find time to write and maybe learn the roads around Seattle, using buses and walking. My fear of driving in big cities with so much stimulus is fed by the bigger fears Jim and I have. I will cope. I have no choice.

The word mortality has nothing to do with length of life, but more to do with living with the fears and the pain and the joy. Already I have had a full life with Jim. He is here for me, and I am here for him. There is no better place to be than where we are.

My next novel deals with "what defines us." I have pondered: Is it where we came from, what we do, how we do it, or what we leave behind? I'll add the ability to give as we receive, and the patience to be present and just be content with what is given, without desire. Finding joy is a choice.

Cancer is never fair. It is not a defining aspect.
Love to all.

∞

April Fools' Day

Easy day when we chose to see the grouse and sun on leaves.
Easy day if we look no farther than the moment.
Easy day with you, even when cancer demands tension.

Email from Teri to Abbe, April 6, 2014

Abbe Dude,

I loved every single word you wrote and cried like a baby after reading your beautiful words. So many different emotions came through, the beauty peeking through the fears, the love piercing through the sadness. Oh, Dude, I love you and am by your side, sending you and Jim the best of my healing thoughts.

Thank you for sharing. I always feel honored to receive anything you write. As I feel honored to be your longtime friend through the highs and lows of beautiful life.

Love you, my strong and courageous friend. Though I've never met Jim, please tell him that, whatever may come, I will always be here for his Abbe.

Love you, Dude,
- Teri

Email from Mary D to Abbe,
April 2014

Hello, my dear friend!

I was just re-reading your first piece and the follow-up essay. I hear Al cursing the tax return in the next room. I went in and told him about Jim's and your journey. He looked at me for a long while and said, "I am such a fool to complain about this." Isn't that the truth!

As I was reading of your experiences in the hospital and at home, the tears were rolling down my cheeks, but I was smiling. I can see you in the story. You have always been a good writer, but that gift has certainly grown and developed into something incredible.
Thank you so much for including me in your journey. Although we are far away, geographically, please know that you are always in my heart and in my thoughts. Sending healing vibes to Jim!

With love,
Mary D

Email from Selma, Abbe's mother, to Jim,
April 10, 2014

Dear Jim,

You bring an abundance of special things into my life. Your warmth and affection to me, and all of the new family you acquired, overwhelms me at times. My comfort and enjoyment with you and Abbe, and seeing your love for each other, are wonderful. You now have

∞

done a first! I have never received a note from a son-in-law. (I think of you as a son.)

Love you and can't wait to see you in May,
- Sel

Email from Selma to Abbe, April 10, 2014

Dear Abbe,

Your loving and beautiful essay, filled with your reality, love, and appreciation of life, touched me so very deeply. My "little bird," you fly like an eagle.

Love you so much,

Mom

Email excerpt from Jim to Tom, May 2, 2014

Hi, Tom,

Regarding this weekend, we have company. The same this afternoon and tonight.

No worries about me, as I progress through the chemo treatments. I'm mostly getting better, lowering the M-spike, and my back hurts less after the radiation. I still have "chemo-brain," I've bulked up in places due to the steroids, and I lack energy.

I'll know more about my schedule in mid-May. Also in

May, my sister-in law and my mother-in law Selma will be here for two weeks. Then if possible, I'd like Selma to spend the better part of the summer here to help Abbe when I have the stem cell transplants in Seattle.

Thanks for keeping in touch. That's all I really need from you and my other friends.
Good to hear your family is doing fine.

- Jim

Email from Jim to family, April 15, 2014

Hi, all.
I've attached a heartfelt e-mail Abbe sent to her family. I place my odds at much better than she does, as I'm going for at least 100 years. Here are my thoughts.

The reason for sending this email is that I will need a bone marrow donor. John had his blood drawn already, but we will need to wait for confirmation from my insurance company to go ahead with the blood analysis to determine if his blood is acceptable.

Please do not think of this as any pressure or to question you if you are not interested in having blood drawn (at your local doctor/clinic), but if John's blood is not a match for me, my best chance of finding the right bone marrow donor is a sibling. Forgive me, but I just need one of you and am having a very difficult time sending this email.

The process is to give blood to determine if it matches me, and that's the easy part. The next phase is to come to

Seattle, check in for several days, and take an injection of a drug that boosts your bone marrow count. Two IVs are then inserted, one in each arm, and you are attached to an apparatus that will filter out the stem cells.

Gracie, I believe your faith does not condone this type of procedure, but I still need to ask. You all will be filling out a form asking personal questions, and someone from SCCA will contact you asking a lot of questions, and that might be another reason to say no.

If you are interested, I can call you to talk this through for the first step.

Thanks,
 Jim

Note from Abbe

Bless your parents.

I believe that the love of your parents created an opportunity for you to thrive. While they lived, they taught and brought a family together. Now in their absence, they have left behind their combined stem cells, their essence, and all your siblings to help each other. You are blessed in so many ways to live, to heal, to experience all the miracles that begin with two cells that combine, two beings, to create intimacy for one and all. I think of freedom, I think of crossing lines of membranes, I think of the right to join, I think of chances and purpose. Bless your parents for their joys in intimacy: Brother Rich is your match!!!!!

Email from Jim to Family,
May 30, 2014

Greetings, All,

The next phase has begun. I call it poked, probed, inspected, and injected.

We checked out of the North Puget Cancer Clinic yesterday and will be checking into the Seattle Cancer Care Alliance next Wednesday the 4th. Now that the plasma cells have been reduced to "all but detectable level," it is time to do the stem cell transplants to get rid of the gene that is causing the havoc. As you know, that means the autologous from me and follow up allogeneic from Richard's stem cells. Just so you know, his process is also grueling, and he'll be in and out of the SCCA mid-August for a week plus. Thank you, Richard.

I begin with a full physical, x-rays, skeletal MRI, EKG, ultrasound of my heart, dental work, dietitian, blah, blah, blah... The installation of a Hickman catheter (surgery for an hour), and then I get my stem cells mobilized, around the 19th of June. This drug, Neupogen, is a protein made with recombinant DNA technology by using E. coli. It will force the cells into the blood and harvest them, which is a four-day process. The same thing happens to Richard. Good luck, Rich. I might get a break to come home right after.

I then get a harsh chemo treatment of Melphalan to rid my body of stem cells and who knows what else such as hair, etc. (Up until now, the treatments have not affected my hair, and I look almost the same.) I then get my stem cells transplanted around the first week of

July. I might need to be hospitalized for a week or so to recuperate. I will be monitored for the next few weeks, and then we begin again.

On or about the second week of August, Rich is admitted and begins with stem cell mobilization, a seven to eleven day process for him. I begin again with the chemo but obviously not the stem cell mobilization, because this time Rich's are injected into me. I also get a full body irradiation to get rid of any last holdouts of the mutant gene. After all of this, I get the stem cell transplant.

Here is where it gets tricky. I need another drug (don't have that name yet) that will help my body "not reject" a foreign body, i.e. Rich's stem cells. I will be closely monitored for the next couple of weeks and loosely monitored for the next three months, taking us into the first part of December. Oh, I also will take periodically a maintenance form of chemo, most likely for the rest of my life, to ensure that if there are any mutant genes lingering around, we keep their count really low.

During this whole time, Abbe will be taking care of me. Thank you, Abbe. We have a condo to stay in, thank you, Janet. Thank you Larry, Steve, and Johnny for volunteering to be a match for me...looks like Richard is the lucky one. My resistance to infection will be greatly lowered, but please keep in touch. Don't know about visitors yet.

That is the short story for my 2014 summer. I know I missed things or got a few dates wrong, and I'm sure the schedule will have modifications. Both Abbe and I will have our laptops and cell phones, and will make it home as often as possible. I will run ATSI, my biological consulting business, but will rely on Karla and Janet to hold down the fort. Thank you, Karla and Janet.

Feel free to share this email.

- Jim

Email from Jim,
June 6, 2014

Hello, All.

Sorry for the broadcast email, but today was long, and so were the previous two. Next week will be intense with SCCA probing me, and basically we do not know what happens (scheduling) beyond a week, not to mention the schedule can change at any time. (An hour ago, they cancelled Sunday's appointment and put one on the docket for Wednesday.) So if you ask us what is going on, we can only provide you with what has happened.

The SCCA team is awesome. Near the end of the coming week, I believe the Violet Team (what they call our team of doctors, nurses, and techs) will meet and say I am ready to begin the transplant process. (I've asked what the color of the team means, fearing that it represented the severity of my cancer, but they have assured me that the colors are random.) The next step depends on what they find inside me. So far, my blood work and response to my chemo ranks at the top of what they have ever seen (seriously) and because brother Richard and I are such a close match in the HLA (a score of 10 out of 10), we are all optimistic. But then I do not gamble.

∞

On Monday, we are meeting with one of the top MM specialists in the world. He is a part of our Violet Team. It's about time the damn stars are aligning for me, since I now have a cancer that affects only 2 percent of the world population (and only 40% of those have the mutant P-53 gene).

Today I had a double bone marrow biopsy. That was it, but dang, it smarted. There are a lot of other issues we are dealing with, but we can discuss that when we see each other. Although there will be times that I will be quarantined, feel free to figure out how to visit us. The condo is small, but the surroundings are large (it is Seattle in Belltown and just north of Pike Place Market).

Note from Abbe

Sunshine in our Souls

I'm not sure how June arrived. Half the year divided, sped-up. One step at a time, the philosophy of recovery to addiction, disease, cancer, life. The pace doesn't matter, just the movement toward a direction. See the broad sweep, distilled down to the minute. Here we are, back six months from Africa. We returned with your crumbling spine, dreams distorted. So many changes. We step forward together. The next leg of the journey is upon us.

Email from Jim,
June 13, 2014

We had an hour question-and-answer conversation with a doctor who specializes in MM. We learned a lot, such as the fact that the autologous transplant isn't really a transplant, but a way to kill all of my bone marrow. In other words, the reason for bone marrow transplants came from strong chemotherapy methods that were used to get rid of cancer. The doctors soon learned that although you can give chemo to a patient to kill the cancer, soon you'd just kill the patient. So the idea is to remove some stem cells, which allows us to kill "all" the bone marrow, and then put the stem cells back in, allowing the patient to live and the cancer to die. A better term for the autologous is "restaging." Transplanting was not the main focus, but a way to kill more potential cancer cells was. Transplanting is a byproduct.

The next treatment, allogeneic, is a true transplant. I go through the chemo (again) and Rich's stem cells get put into me...thus the transplant. Rich, I'd like to sit with you to go over what I learned that you will be experiencing. Thanks again for volunteering.

John, because of timing issues and the need to have a "second caregiver for a backup," I need to talk with you about taking care of me if Abbe cannot (sickness, other commitments).

The only reason for my allogeneic stem cell transplant is primarily because of the mutant gene. That damn mutant gene is rearing its ugly head (I will learn more about it in the next few weeks).

∞

Larry, the mutant gene issue is particular to my form of MM. What happens with MM in general is that a small portion of a particular gene, and there are at least 10 variants of said gene, controls the production of plasma cells. I have, on top of the basic form of MM, a mutant gene. The MM gene that is stuck in the "on" position is typical of most MM patients. My mutant gene is atypical and is stuck on the "off" position. The mutant gene is hard to find in our bodies and generally only observed with a more intensive blood analysis. Also, MM in general is not typically found in "other family members." So for now, I do not believe that any of my other family members or even relatives have anything to worry about because I have the disease. It is not hereditary. If you are truly concerned, I recommend you talk with a knowledgeable doctor, have a blood draw, and look for the M-spike and/or do a biopsy of your bone marrow and check for elevated levels of plasma cells. But before you go through that expense, let me know: I will connect you with my doctor, and he will consult with you appropriately.

**Email from Abbe to Frances,
June 15, 2104**

You know you are a writer and a comedian when you are given news that is considered "sobering," and all you can think is that you want a glass or two or three of wine. Eventually I'll write the essay, the joke, the funny story, but today I'll just send you an update. Jim and I putter in our Seattle condo, each of us with our offices set up in our one room. Desks facing the window, sofa facing the TV with few channels, dining table facing the kitchen. It is called two-step living. We do this well. Here is the latest.

∞

Yesterday was a reality check with the doctors. The cancer trials offered have less than optimal results. We are working against odds. Remission for a longer period than five years seems to be elusive. Also, Jim has more fractures in his spine, and the percentage of myeloma in his plasma has risen to 4%, not unexpected, but it shows the aggression of the cancer cells. After a good night of sleep, we are back in the saddle, doing all the protocols. Jim is no longer drinking wine and is not to lift anything. Walking is a mandate, as is hydration and staying healthy.

All in life is good, and Jim and I love the life we live.

**Email from Frances to Abbe,
June 16, 2014**

Dear Abbe,

You know you are a writer when you set up a desk in a temporary apartment south of home. And write about suffering while including a joke. I think of you often and send you and Jim love, good thoughts, and hope (*speranza* sounds better) as you travel through these coming weeks.

Take care, much love to both of you,
- Frances

Cocoon of Cancer

Jim snores, curled up on an opened futon in our one-room condo, wrapped in a black, comfy blanket, dressed to leave. He meant just to take a break, a pause, after eating his daily cup of pills and drinking a spot of water. He meant to drink his peanut power smoothie, but instead he snores curled in sleep.

The other day he looked at me with eyes watered with sincerity. "Tell me, Abbe, how is it that I feel closer to you now? I never felt closer to anyone before, and now I feel closer?"

I smiled and wrapped his hand in my palm. "I know. This is the best."

Perhaps the answer lies within perpetual making of love, the simmered smooth actions of deep affection. After Jim received his over-the-top chemotherapy, a drug called Melphalan, with warnings on the label, use only once in a lifetime, and then his infusions of his own stem cells, an odd smell encircled the room. DMSO, a preservative for stem cell freezing and also a liniment for horses, wafted through Jim's system and out his mouth and through his sweat. Only some people are lucky enough to have a gene that controls this odor. That night I insisted on spooning, so that either way we slept, his breath was opposite mine. Loving the feel of Jim, my arms encircled him. His body twisted to hold me with his legs.

I've come to label this new adventure "the cocoon of cancer." Jim, with his two tattoos, smiles at the

∞

analogy. His tiger swallowtail butterfly on one arm, his frog on the other, symbolize the metamorphosis of life. Our cocoon envelops cancer patients, medical teams, and caregivers. There is no guarantee of remission. Jim won't sprout wings but will have permanent outward changes. Inside the cocoon we go inward, changing how we view life. Those within the cocoon embody all ages, all nationalities, and all sizes.

You begin to recognize individual faces after the daily ritual of blood draws. You can hear each patient spell their name, repeat their birthday to the attending nurse. In my sleep I repeat Jim's response. J A M E S R O B E R T W I G G I N S   JUNE 11, 1951.   Each procedure, each attending physician, each action is met with verification. If you didn't know who you were before, you know now.

Anonymous faces tell you stories. You discern if they are beginners in this journey. They hold their schedules tight, they come in with wide eyes. Those farther along nod acknowledgment of your presence. And those in the midst of chemo or transplant shuffle in, give a weary smile, or hold their breath, hoping to have enough energy to walk, sit, and not vomit. Some have legs swollen with regimen-related toxicities, others sport new headdresses. You see the tears, fears, hopes in all the faces. They are one. They are Jim now and later.

Jim still dresses fashionably. But now he makes sure his pants are loose around the waist, that he has layers to ward off the chill, and a shirt that opens easily to access his Hickman catheter. His father's hand-carved, diamond-willow cane is a new accessory to and from the car. Inside the clinic, my arm presses into his body. I feel his warmth, he feels my steadying pace.

Like most of the patients at Seattle Cancer Care Alliance, we are physically away from home. I think that is what it should be. Our true home has nothing to do with doctors and illness, at least we hope not. Living in a condo in a busy metropolis, far from our twenty acres, we create rituals, knitting a city home, darning the holes to keep us secure.

Jim and I adapt. Instead of a nice walk down our quarter-mile driveway, we push "L" for lobby and check the mailbox. Even our stance has changed. Jim has shrunk from 5'9" to 5'6". His present stature brings him in closer to my 4'11" (or maybe 4'10.5"). I still stretch upward on my toes for a kiss, finding a new nook to hold his arm, but with the change in height all his pants hit the floor. One afternoon, after a reality talk from our medical team, Jim asks me to find a tailor. I jump at the chance, anything to run from the grim prognosis and statistics that the doctors must declare. With a plastic garbage bag in hand, I enter a tailor shop on the corner of Wall and Third Avenue, a two-block walk from our condo. The owner greets me and asks me what I need. Words stick in my throat, as I pull out an old khaki pair of pants with the inseam of the crotch torn, a pair of new pants, and an old red and blue plaid shirt with a blown-out elbow. The Korean owner waits as tears roll down my face. My hands shake and I'm embarrassed at my loss of composure, the cocoon ripping at the edge. Finally I blurt out, "My husband has cancer and he is shorter, the pants are longer, and this is his favorite shirt. Can you help me?"

To a stranger I pour out my tears. She holds my hand, tells me that the shirt is very hard to fix. I say okay, forget the shirt. But she insists, "If this is your husband's favorite shirt, I will fix it. He must have it. I will fix it cheap." I find out that she, too, is in the cocoon. Her husband died of cancer two years past, and she knows the importance of the shirt.

Relevance, normalcy, routine, protocol, elevators, appointments, eating, bathing; all become the rituals we cling to in order to transform into a new way of life. Jim, who loves to cook and savor flavors, has not eaten in a week. The chemotherapy Melphalan kills his stem cells, gradually depleting the counts of his remaining white, red, and platelet cells. While his newly-infused stem cells try to find their way back to the bone marrow and begin new growth, his body reacts with nausea, sloughing off the old cells in a gastro dance from the mouth to the bottom. Everyone says he is doing well. He is in day four of his rebirth (day one they call his birthday). If Jim survives the dying, we will celebrate three birthdays this year. The one he repeats daily to the staff, June 11, 1951; July 14, the day his own stem cells infused; and sometime in the next month, another birthday when he receives his brother Richard's stem cells.

I miss eating with Jim. Our pattern of cooking together dissolves. I resort to my old recipes of stir-fries and layered salads. But there is no comfort in eating alone, no joy, just the knowledge that I have to eat so that I am able to be there with Jim. And we still snuggle on the couch, after I have sterilized the kitchen, made all safe for Jim's weakened immune system. I don't really need to re-heat three of my homemade frozen cookies

∞

each night. But Jim and I both know that this is another attempt at affection. My treats become our treats as we hold fast to the evening, watching mysteries on PBS.

Jim is skinny. I watch his square shoulders, wider than any shoulders I have ever seen, carry his head forward, his legs straggling behind, as he concentrates on moving. If I ask too many times, "What can I get for you?" his response is quick, sharp, "Make the next five days go quicker. Get this over with."

I wish I could. Instead I bring him another juice to drink, make sure he has had the correct pills. I learn to clean and flush his Hickman catheter, and then I learn to infuse him with liquids. I may be nursing him, but I am not a nurse. When I wrap his port for a shower, I watch him leave me. I take time to memorize his back, butt, legs, and shoulders. I get the benefit of kissing his chest, and when I stop and kiss the top of his head, Jim leans into my breasts and plants a kiss.

Today he sleeps and visits the bathroom. Food is a struggle. He warns me that tomorrow he might have to go the hospital, if he can't eat or drink. His brother John will be here, as I'm off to visit my daughter Mara. Mara carries a new life within her, and I want to dissuade her fears, calm her nerves, and be part of this future. All the while, Jim wants not to fear, to have all the burdens removed. I understand, but fear has left me. I want only the tenderness of being close.

I listen to the news, all sad. The plane over the Ukraine shot down by insurgents, the Israel and Palestine fight on the Gaza Strip, the hotbeds of hatred and judgment that miss life altogether. Here at the Seattle Cancer

Care Alliance, the international world walks within the cancer cocoon. Patients travel from England, India, Russia, and from across all oceans for care. Compassion meets eye-to-eye, tears fall, we smile, bump knuckles, pat hands, share conversations.

Jim asks me if he will ever leave the cocoon of cancer. I don't have an answer with so many procedures to come, so many statistics of remission quoted. I believe he will be healthier, get strong, eat and drink with me again. I will curl inside his heart and he into mine. I promise him intimacy.

The Seattle Cancer Alliance keeps us informed. Their tentative schedule outlines the next leg of our journey. Four months in local treatment by our home and then this will be our life in Seattle. Procedures vary with Jim's unexpected physical issues but for the most part the schedule holds true. Once involved in the program, we have a daily and weekly calendar. Our time belongs to cancer.

SCCA Tentative Schedule:

June 4—Sixth floor History and Physical at 12:45 pm. First floor blood draw at 1:30 pm. Meet team Violet, Molly
June 5—Appointment not set yet
June 6—Possible bone marrow biopsy

June 9 to 13
Bone skeletal X-rays and MRI
Urine collection 24 hours (checks kidney function)
Heart monitoring   (EKG-Echo test)
Lungs/Chest X-ray, Pulmonary functions
Dental exam and cleaning
Meet Pharmacist/Dietician/Social Worker
Caregiver classes (now or later)

June 16 to 20
Prepare for Hickman catheter
June 18—Surgery 45-90 minutes
June 19—Start mobilization of stem cells. (Uses one drug, Neupogen protein, to grow stem cells and crowd out other cells. Three hours each day to filter for 4 days: 19 to 22. Will feel bone achiness, flu-like symptoms)

June 25 to 27—Potentially go home
June 30—Monday chemo 30 to 60 minutes, Melphalan

(most likely this harsher chemo will knock Jim out)
July 2—Stem cell transplant
July 7 to 20—Side effects: spiked fever, sore mouth, wiped out. If admitted to UW hospital, 2 to 4 weeks. Abbe can stay 24/7
July 21—Discharge Jim back to condo. Abbe takes over managing fluids and medicine. (Three to four weeks)
This takes 42 days total.

August 12—Brother Richard begins stem mobilization
Jim has full body irradiation, 15 to 20 minutes
August 16 to 20—Second stem cell transplant
100 days of monitoring

50/50 chance of engrafting/hosting complication
Home by end of November/ beginning of December

Email from Jim, First week of July, 2014

Time for Tissues.

Here's my version of the past ten days, a short story. Before I begin this recent account, just so you know, all is well and going as planned. We are both optimistic about the outcome of the tandem transplant and my going into remission post-therapy. Seems like we are on an unbroken horse. Sometimes it's a wild ride and other times it's just a buddy taking us on its journey, but the horse is in charge. All we do is hang on.

My back (two lumbar and three thoracic vertebrae) is broken from the myeloma, and it remains sore. I have an appointment with an orthopedic surgeon at Group Health on Wednesday to discuss surgery. I am looking forward to that, even though I have always told myself I'd never have surgery on my back. From what I understand, the kyphoplasty procedure is an injection of a cement substance that will create space between my collapsed vertebrae and shore up the fractures. I'm game for this, as the pain slows me down, preventing a normal routine through the day.

On the 20th of June I began the Neupogen injections to mobilize my stem cells to prepare for apheresis. Twice a day for three days (trips back and forth to the SCCA) with side effects of fatigue and bone pain. Pain similar to that of growing pains of a child who suddenly has a two-inch growth spurt. I mostly slept and didn't eat much. Since I'm still trying to get my pain meds figured out, the physical pain drains me and knocks me out. I take Tramadol and acetaminophen. On Monday I had apheresis, where both ports of my Hickman are hooked up to a machine that draws the blood out. Centrifugal force separates the blood, and the stem cells are harvested. The goal for the autologous transplant was 10 million cells per kg of body weight. An appointment was made for Tuesday because we assumed that since my stem cell production had been slow the first two days, I would not make that goal. The SCCA would let us know by 4:30 pm, because if we did not harvest 10 million cells I needed to get another Neupogen shot in the early evening. We finished up after five hours and went back to the condo.

I got a call around 4:00 pm, and the person said they harvested 87 million cells. Holy crap, I hit the jackpot....

But that sounded too strange and I questioned the results, as it seemed implausible, given all the circumstances, that it could be this high.

We had an appointment the following day with our nurse, the physician's assistant (PA), and our doctor. I asked them, so what does 87 million mean? Although they all questioned the high number and the PA contacted the lab with questions, the lab said, "Hey, we ran the analysis and that's the number, no need to question us." Our doctor said I have a strong and healthy bone marrow to produce that high a number. With this news, Abbe and I felt pretty good and had an understanding that my body was doing quite well, and we could move forward with the first phase of the transplant with a healthy supply of stem cells. Although I still did not truly understand what 87 million meant, I just accepted the analysis of the lab. Since we had a little "free time," we planned on a long weekend back home.

∞

On Thursday evening around 7:00 pm, my doctor called. My cell phone was busy, so he called Abbe's. He stated to her that he had bad news (not something to tell anyone with cancer, or the caregiver without an explanation). I grabbed her phone and talked with the doctor, and he stated that the lab had made a mistake. They only harvested 3 million stem cells. He stated they could work with that number, but a minimum of 10 million would be best. He apologized several times and said the SCCA would cover these extra costs. I remained calm and discussed with him when to reschedule or restart the mobilization process with Neupogen shots and another session of apheresis. Because we planned on heading home, I had scheduled a business meeting on Monday. Because July 4th is a holiday and the weekend, new injections for the mobilization would have to be postponed until Monday the 7th and set our time back another week because the SCCA does not do apheresis on the holidays.

Well, you can't say that to Abbe and get away with it. The following day when I was in physical therapy, Abbe met with our nurse. Her meeting was about our disappointment with protocol, questioning how a prestigious clinic like the SCCA could make such a mistake/miscalculation. Not to mention, how could our team not realize that 87 million was not even close to the normal results of my type of apheresis and use some clout to question the results? According to Abbe, the conversation was heartfelt and serious. Abbe and our nurse held hands as they talked. She expressed her disappointment with the apheresis and analysis sections of the SCCA, knowing how painful it had been for me. Abbe emphasized the need to understand the lab's culture of denial and why no one spotted the red flags. Abbe also requested the mobilization process be started as soon as we returned, stating that "cancer does not take a holiday."

What bothers us most is how this mistake happened, and the fact I need to go through another three-day session of bone pain. I will survive this, as I know what is coming, and was able to deal with it once already. Regardless, I do need to start over. The other and most critical concern is, if someone in the lab had not finally questioned the 87 million in the analysis section and not retested my apheresis results, and if we had moved forward with the chemo portion and the autologous phase, and they needed 4 million instead of the 3 million stem cells they had, I could have died. Or if the stem cell transplant from Richard failed, I would have no reserves and then most likely would die. The hospital term for this mistake is a "near miss." "Near misses" are cause for an internal investigation.

On Friday afternoon, Abbe got a call from the medical director of the lab as well as apheresis. He called to apologize and to let us know that an investigation had been launched, from the technician to every step on the analysis. Abbe requested to be on the team of resolution and discovery, again stating that "cancer does not take a holiday," not the 4th of July nor weekends. The doctor promised her that the lab would be open for us and that a meeting of all our team, including him, would be scheduled next week. So we now return to Seattle and begin the mobilization of my stem cells on Wednesday, with apheresis on Saturday. Hopefully we will work something out with my spine, and I can begin the chemo and autologous transplant the beginning of next week.

- Jim

∞

Note from Abbe to Jim

Have you ever climbed up a slope to a pinnacle to see an incredible site, and below lies a green-blue pool of water, the swimming hole for locals? This is the jump spot where everyone leaps to the bottom. You come to the edge and peer down. You look over to see if there are rocks in your way. You calculate the angle and distance from the rock face to set you free. That leap of faith, the release of letting go, pulls, but you hold back. You go down a foot, then a yard, to steal more time and recalculate. People below call out and look up at you. All wait for the plunge. Why jump? Why stay? Is it faith, wisdom, need, choice? Free falling.

Email from Abbe to Shannon at Robeks Corporation, July 12, 2014

We have been in Seattle since June 4th. Jim has had every test imaginable to make sure his body can withstand the demands of a tandem cell transplant. We have a medical team that monitors Jim's progress. The Hickman catheter installed in his chest saves him from much prodding and poking and will allow for the exit and entrance of the stem cells. When we don't have to go to the labs at Seattle Cancer Care Alliance, I clean and flush out the Hickman tubes. I've had to put aside my fears of driving in the big city, my discomfort in hospitals, and queasiness at the sight of blood. I've been in every procedure with Jim: spinal taps (looks like a maple tree giving up its syrup), bone marrow extractions, and chemo infusions. Somehow we have forged a union that elevates us into a more intimate sharing. The medical team picks up on this and responds with more openness.

∞

I have only been able to return to my Robeks café and our home twice. We have elicited help from friends and family, and they keep a watch on the essentials. Let Robeks Corporation know that Jim has a Peanut Power smoothie every day with Greek yogurt and whey protein. He can't have the vitamins or the probiotics due to contraindications with his medicines and immune system. When he is ill, and this will be truer after the next round of chemo and radiation, the smoothie might be his only food. I have friends picking the smoothies up frozen, and carting them off to Seattle when they come to visit.

Best to all the staff,
- Abbe

**Email excerpt from Shannon to Abbe,
July 12, 2014**

I shared your e-mail with the staff at Robeks. It is amazing what we can endure for the ones we love. I guess sometimes, through tough times, we recognize strengths we never knew existed. Sounds like you have faced those fears and run right through them.

Jim is a rock star in my book. I admire his fight, courage, and strength.

- Shannon

Email from Abbe to family,
July 13, 2014

Jim is sucking ice, has been since 8:30 a.m. The chemo Melphalan is now in his system, and we will remain in the infusion ward at SCCA until about 3:00 PM for hydration and flushing out Jim's system. Surreal, with all the bags hanging on a pole, tubes extending into his Hickman catheter, and computers beeping orders.

Our spirits are high, knowing how much you all care. Monday is day zero, when we return for eight hours for his stem cell infusion, Jim's reboot.

Email from Laurie to Abbe,
July 13, 2014

Good Morning, Abbe,

Wow, my heart is so heavy after reading your essays. You are such an incredible writer in the midst of all of this chaos. I would have no words, and you are so eloquent in describing yours and Jim's despair. Jim is so lucky to have you, and of course the love you have for him shines through all this craziness.

I have been in your restaurant many times, and the staff seem to be doing just fine. They are always courteous and efficient and whip up cool, delicious treats. Your ten years of connecting with the community will not fall apart during these next months. I know December must feel like an eternity to you. I am always happy to visit Robeks, and I will make a point to frequent it more often and let you know if I notice anything out of the ordinary. If you need anything else, Steve and I would be honored to help you both. We are here for you in heart and spirit through this journey. Love to you both.

- Laurie

Email from Abbe to Laurie,
July 15, 2014

My intent certainly wasn't to weigh your heart down, just the opposite. Within all the despair, there remains the pair, Jim and I. Distilled down to what we value and what we can create. Just this morning, I rose at 4:00 am and had a great yoga session, and because there is a pool where we are staying, I swam for a delightful half-hour. Jim woke and we tried to shave his head. I got halfway through and the shaver broke. Jim, half-shaved, showered. Afterwards, I hooked him up to the pump for his saline solution infusion, and now he is asleep. We laugh because we can. When Jim awakens, he'll look in the mirror. There is always a hat.

We are on day eight since the transplant. The bewitching day of stem cell regenerations is just a few days away. Without a fever, Jim remains out of the hospital, but eating will be the key. So far nothing works. Good thing I'm not sensitive about my cooking.

Laurie, Jim and I both value our friends, small gestures, laughing, and finding joy in what makes the world comfortable. No greed in any of this. So my heart is not heavy, in fact it is lighter with new understanding. Thanks for your kind words, energy, and all that you are.

Celebrate each moment.

Love,
Abbe

Email from Jan to Abbe and Jim,
July, 2014

We are in Courtney, BC, celebrating our anniversary. I didn't feel comfortable leaving. When you get a chance, will you update us about how things are going? Our compromise is that we can come back any time if things get bad for you. Johnny roasted chicken pieces for Jim on Monday. We will bring them down next week.

Much love to you both,
Jan

Email from Abbe to Jan and John,
July, 2014

I'm so glad you and Johnny got away to your summer music concert and are able to celebrate your anniversary. Even when there are tough times for loved ones, your mom and Jim, you need to relax and revitalize the self. I can picture you and Johnny helping with the set-up, enjoying friends and music. Nice.

Jim did well this last round of mobilization. He took more medication and was able to weather most of the effects of bone pain and fatigue. Sunday and Monday were the hardest, but he is able to eat now. He finally figured out that part of his problem was nausea and that he can take a prescription for that. You can't always identify what is going on. The learning curve is steep.

Will took me grocery shopping today. Fun stuff. I can remember shopping with Will when he was a little boy. His curiosity then overwhelmed me, but today he made my life simple.

∞

Saturday begins the next phase. Day zero is considered the first day of transplant. From what we have learned, the third day might be the most difficult, but gradually it gets better, with most people feeling okay by day ten. Our medical team will monitor Jim to make sure he is doing well. Check in with us/me, so I can hear your voice. Our goal is to stay hydrated, with no fever, and to have the white blood count return to normal after transplant. If there are any problems, Jim will be sent to the University of Washington Medical Center.

You guys are rock solid, the best family and friends anyone could have.

Love,
Abbe

Email from Abbe to Harriet,
July 13, 2014

Good morning, Har,

I've been up since four this morning, in search of a serene slice of calm. Not that the other moments are hectic, only that they carry demand, fears, and observations. Moments of vigilance.

Jim is holding down some food, smoothies, yogurt, and hopefully some scrambled eggs. He quells the queasy feelings with difficulty, experimenting with different anti-nausea pills. I know the sensation way too well, and wish I could switch bodies as my body has learned the signs and what to do. Jim is the investigator and needs to learn first-hand. I hold his hand as he finds

∞

his way. Showered and now resting, Jim will make his daily trip to SCCA with me later this morning. The center's system of daily visits works as a great way to watch over patients.

I've washed two loads of laundry so far. When we return, I'll scrub the kitchen and bathrooms with bleach and then the bedroom shades and anything we touch (TV clicker, light switches, computers). Jim is susceptible to all bacteria.

The sun shines, the temperature has already risen to seventy. I'm itching to write something significant.

Love you,
Abbe

More Sharp Bends in the Road

Sometime during the month of July, my mother started to worry about Jim. Her stomach hurt. She dismissed the signs as anxiety. She finally went to the doctors, and they gave her the diagnosis of pancreatic cancer. Between all of Jim's procedures, I traveled back and forth to Palm Springs and then to Los Angeles to be there for her. Her cancer progressed quickly, and she passed over to another world in November. Along the way, I kept her aware of Jim's struggle to survive.

Email from Abbe to Jim, July 30, 2014

(I'm in Palm Springs with Mom)

I tried to sleep in this morning, although we didn't turn in until 10:30 pm. My mom sleeps with her bedroom TV on all night, and the sounds migrate my way. Not as bad as the over-zealous partiers and homeless street people outside our Seattle condo window, but I imagine she has been doing this since before my dad passed away. Voices make her feel less lonely, console her in some way that allows her to sleep.

We have had some "giveaway" talks, and I can see her dilemma with always trying to make things "even" not only for Harriet and me, but for her grandkids. She tries to weigh things in her mind with a bias unbeknownst to her, of how she views our wants and desires. She has a difficult job. Her treasures live on.

∞

I do believe she will not take any medications, not opt for the Gemzar drug and only deal with constipation, nausea, and pain. She worries about leaving Harriet, and puts me firmly by your side. She lives vicariously through our love story and wants to keep that alive. I tell her about our tender times when the world swirls around us and we lie on the futon watching TV, holding hands. My romance becomes hers, and she believes few have achieved the depth and softness that you and I have. She is correct. I think in a way that is our gift to her.

My mom has an elegance, a sophistication, all the way down to her toes. Her roots want to laugh and be silly. Her shoe fetish began as a child. She sold shoes at one of her early jobs, and just last month she bought a beautiful pair of suede strapped shoes with a low heel, at a cost of $200, now never worn. She would like to return them, because the season for their wearing won't come soon enough for her life span. She closes the shoe box wistfully. I look at my feet, trying to elongate them from a size 5.5 to 8.5. Walking in her shoes would be nice.

Email from Abbe to Jim,
August 14, 2014

Even as I have been here for less than one day, my mom says she feels the deterioration, the change in her condition. She felt queasy and had a bowl of ice cream. She is resting. I'm not sure how to describe her stomach, GI tract, and sense of malaise. I watch, knowing your journey from the first stem cell transplant. You are on the upswing to heal, and she is on the downswing, uncomfortable with sensations that rob her. Dis-ease. I don't think she wants to pretend. She wants the end to be swift. I don't know if that will be possible. She rests on the sofa in the den, wrapped in a blanket, her hair twisted in a leftover bun from the day before. I know too much and not enough....

On August 20ᵗʰ, Paige was born to my daughter Mara and her husband AJ. Paige arrived three weeks early. Mara went into labor when Jim and I were in a meeting with the new medical team, the Red Team, in charge of Jim's allogeneic transplant. There was a pause, then cries of joy and wonder.

Email from Abbe to Jim, August 20, 2014

When a baby comes into this world, their innocence opens everyone's heart. The miracle suspends judgment on worthiness. The baby comes with a clean slate, and their life depends on those who surround them with warmth, sustenance, and gentle care. Their basic needs are fulfilled easily, and rewards come by way of smiles and coos.

When a person of age leaves this world, hearts are heavy, and simplicity, now complicated by competing desires, fills the slate. A cloud of expectations rains over every decision, as the voice of the dying echoes. Warmth, sustenance, gentle care are complicated by pain, and the living's desires stacked in sloppy piles of well-meaning intentions.

Birth and death, both part of the cycle of life, belabored with time.

Nine months to create, and the indefinite question mark of exit.

Birth presents a future. Death erases a past.

Voices clamor for attention.

The cries of innocence proceed.

The wails of judgment recede.

One life lived with love

peels back the essence.

Sweet smiles reflect

on those who remain.

Earth's Rotation

Jim and I find the seasons changing from the muggy heat of city reflections to crisp evenings and darkened mornings. The earth rotates as we find our balance in our cancer home in Seattle. Tethered by schedules, we follow the protocols of our treatment trial. From Jim's rebirth, his auto stem cell transplant on July 14, 2014, till day forty, we stay within the ten-minute requisite range, only slipping home when our schedule has a window of two days without consultations or tests.

On one of these days at home, I walk along our country road, early before the rooster crows. The neighbor's horses lazily eat in their corralled roundabout. Molly the black lab watches as I pass, no longer running and barking at my intrusion into her space, perhaps a sign I have not been forgotten. The five pugs run along the fence, circling like their curled tails. The only person I know awake at this hour is a longtime friend in Florida. I call and we stroll on a virtual walk as we philosophize about life, pain, and love. I share with her a consoling sense of peace that my own mother is so vital, powerful, and alive. I thank the stars for her support.

Then a star slips and cascades through the sky with a diagnosis of stage four pancreatic cancer. The unthinkable journey of two of my beloved encircles my heart. Selma, my mother, age 86, starts on another trajectory around this planet, her pain heightened by the sadness that she will leave me alone to face Jim's journey, that she will miss the adult grandchildren's bright spirits, their surprises.

Never once do I falter and think that some awful trick

∞

has been played, that the world has a cruel edge. I find my heels edging the ground, my roots powering through the earth's crust, willing myself to flourish, to grow tall with all that lies before me.

As Jim heals, stealing himself for his next round of procedures, I again slip away to visit my mother in Palm Springs. Stark mountains rise with their ripples near her home, burnished by the wind, tooled by water and weathering time. I meet my sister Harriet there, where we luxuriate in our mother's home of thirty-some years. With the inevitable end in sight, our Mom parcels out her jewels, decides on her fate, and secures her daughters' and grandchildren's future. The planner, the financier, the rock of the family, she wears her ripples with pride. Her bucket list won't be complete unless she can see Jim again, and her grandchildren.

Fifty days after Jim's first stem cell transplant, my mother travels with my sister Harriet for a week visit. Between this visit and my visit to the desert, another star has twinkled in the sky. Paige Selma Porter arrived three weeks early. Mara, my eldest daughter, has carried this bundle of joy through a thirty-six week pregnancy mired with nausea that mimicked Jim's. I hold in my arms new life, the future, the legacy of my mother. Paige combines all that was and would be more. We relay our stories of Grandma Sel, now Great Grandma Sel, Gigi Sel, and explain why she held the honored name of Selma.

Now my mom's visit to Seattle has come and gone. Most days she rallied to join in the festivities. Cancer held her tight with pain in the mornings, and still she teased her gray hair into a bun, donned her makeup,

∞

dressed in grays, black, and white. She'd swing her legs over the arm of a chair, a comfort habit that revealed her sense of irony, elegance, and simplicity. Her bucket list overflowed with family. Jim's brothers Rich and John, with their wives Shirley and Jan, were here to support Jim in his next stem cell transplant, and they showered her with well-deserved love. Their genuine friendship celebrated all life.

The day Mom returns to her Palm Springs home, the earth turns back to Jim's trajectory. Wednesday, September 10, 2014, Jim receives his brother Rich's stem cells. This rebirth feels old, tired and strained. Jim's body, worn from past chemo treatments, the march of his own stem cells barely mature, still struggles with his ravaged skeleton. The multiple myeloma, down to a miniscule dot, has left its mark. Richard passes three days in mobilization. His labor of love pushes his body to the max, leaving him low in platelets and in danger of internal bleeding. The first two harvests fall short of the 5 million mark, and with much debate, three doctors confer and decide that with care, Rich could harvest again.

As Rich harvests, Jim receives total body irradiation and two bags of Rich's stem cells, a total of 3.8 million. Determined not to fail his younger brother, Rich turns his system on end to right Jim's system, and on his third try arrives at the miracle number. Without enough stem cells, Jim's own immune system would wipe out Richard's stem cells. The goal of eventual peace, a truce between two systems, is Richard's strong stem cells ridding Jim of the last of the myeloma.

Today is day four. Jim rests now. All families have

returned home. Although it is quiet, I still feel the devotion of Rich and Shirley, John and Jan. Their presence reverberates through the halls of the Seattle Cancer Care Alliance. Smiles, hugs, resemblances shadow our path. One staff member gave Jim her Celtic knot necklace to wear during the stem cell transplant. We share the circle of life—the energy of rebirth, the closeness we all feel to this edge.

I've been here before with Jim, who sleeps most of the day. I remember the hydration overcome by nausea, the pill regime, and the infusions. I'm no longer a newbie. I call the SCCA, I infuse, and I refuse to waver. For the next one hundred days I will lie beside Jim in the curve of his back, my belly abutted. I'll massage the broken spine, I'll smile into his deep blue eyes. Hairless, he shines through with his curious nature. I expect to see the Wiggins' will, now fortified in blood. I straddle the needs of my loves. Just as I feel in the presence of my mother and my first grandchild, I know the world will continue to spin, and we can be assured that their and Jim's indomitable wills match that of gravity.

And when the moment is ripe, we'll toe dance within the circle of life.

**Email from Abbe to Cheryll and Gary,
September 8, 2014**

We are in the midst of the transplant process. The incredible support of Rich and John and Shirley and Jan makes our life easier. Rich has gone through two rounds of apheresis, and today will be the third. Jim received total body irradiation yesterday, and two rounds of stem cells from Rich. He is exhausted. The devotion and love emanated so strongly from our group that the halls of the SCCA felt our presence. One staff member gave Jim her Celtic knot necklace to wear during the transplant. It represents the circle of life, the energy of rebirth, and the closeness we all feel to this edge.

My mom is back home now and will move in with Harriet next week. She brought to all of us the elegance of a proud woman who celebrates. She gave us energy.

Cheryll, teaching is such a hard job. You are a trainer of the next generation. That makes me smile. Gary, Happy Birthday. Enjoy camping.

- Abbe

**Email from Teri to Abbe,
September 9, 2014**

Hi, Abbe Dude,

We are back home from our Seattle visit. Tom and I felt so much strength coming from you in every which way, and we marveled at how our longtime buddy could be so wise and amazingly present, touching life at its core, seeing the beauty amidst the pain. I realize that this is who you have always been for me. The one friend more than any other who truly does touch life and experiences how very precious it is. Hi to Jim. Please let him know how happy we were to finally meet the man who makes our dude glow so brightly.

- Teri

Email from Jim,
September 24, 2014

Hello all, here's an update.

Positive progress to my getting better has been slow and sure.

First and foremost, I feel well, better than I have for quite some time. Second, my feet hurt, swollen from the side effects of the Cyclosporine, which is one of the two drugs (Mycophenolate mofetil/MMF the other) that are T-cell inhibitors to prevent and treat GVHD. My hands also shake, my blood pressure is up, and I have spots in front of my eyes at times, but my hair is finally growing back, what's left of it.

The purpose of these two heavy-duty drugs is to reduce my immunity to allow Rich's stem cells to settle into my body. That's the entire purpose of the second phase, allogeneic, of this tandem transplant. I am feeling well now and getting better as each day passes. I am eating better, and gaining some weight, not too much as I am now three inches shorter than when this all began. This height and weight is the new normal for me. The good news is I can fit into all those clothes that were getting tight around the waist but I had not thrown away.

I slowly crawl out of this hole called cancer, being helped tremendously by Abbe, to remember all the pills, which order and when to swallow them, and to question the clinic staff of their purpose. She is saving my life. And of course thanks to Richard for his stem cells that will soon become a part of me. Their job is to rid my body of all multiple myeloma cells because those are the foreign cells my stem cells still recognize as "me" that Richard's stem cell won't recognize and therefore will do what an immune system is supposed to do, rid my body of this foreign substance. At least that is the theory. This transfer from my stem cells with Richard's is a slow process. They "find" their way into my marrow and settle in. All the while, through blood tests and bone marrow biopsies, the team modulates the immune suppressant drugs I am consuming, and then eventually weans me off of them.

But the possibility of graft versus host disease lingers in my body. That's where the donor cells become aggressive and attack more than just the myeloma, such as my gut or skin. Thus the reason for all the meds, blood tests, and constantly modifying my regime to keep up with the transplant and how my body is responding. My job is to stay healthy and to recognize when I am not healthy. Sounds both stupid and simple, but it is a tough job because I do not feel normal and have not since last November. John and Richard call me "bubble boy" because right now and for another month, until Rich's stem cells begin producing blood (white blood cells), I am highly susceptible to infection. They say this vulnerability could last a year.

∞

The autologous process, my first stem cell transplant about 65 days ago with the melphalan chemo, was very harsh on my entire system, as it brought me to the edge of death. It was intended to do that, so recovery took a while. I was nauseated and could not drink fluids, so food would not stay down and I lost 15 pounds. Most people go into the hospital during this time, but because I was not running a fever, and I stayed "healthy," I stayed out of the hospital, which was a good thing.

After that 65 days of recovery, Richard came into my life, literally. The tests showed no indication of MM in my body, but flow cytometry indicated a 0.0028 percent of the M-spike that is an indicator of the mutant P-53 gene. I realize that is not the best of news, but these treatments are slowly knocking back all semblance of MM and therefore being effective.

Moving onto where we are today, I must emphasize that I feel good in terms of where I am in the protocol. The total body irradiation before Rich's stem cell transplant wasn't as harsh as my first chemo treatment, but the effects linger. I am now eating regularly, although small meals because my stomach shrank as did my bladder. I am being infused with a saline solution daily (I have a portable pump) and drink as much liquids as possible to flush my kidneys as well as my blood stream, to assist in passing the MM out of my body. Most of the symptoms such as high blood pressure come from the 32 pills I take daily. All is temporary. Abbe and I have had the luxury of visiting our new grandchild. Paige and I have much in common. She is one month old, and my new system is just 13 days old. We eat, sleep, rest, heal, grow, and rediscover.

We are beginning to plan more trips to see the world, that's how optimistic we are.

Take care, see your doctor regularly, ask a lot of questions, and stay healthy.

- Jim

**Email from Abbe to Jim,
October 4, 2014**

I'm up late, corrupted by my mom, watching romantic movies.

Harriet and Steve came home a few minutes ago. Mom felt better for a while and now has disappeared into her bed. As she sat reading, her beauty struck me. I told her how beautiful she was and she smiled shyly and then told me she'd hug that thought in bed. More than once she told me how special it was, doing nothing with me. I concurred.

So happy that you and John are together. Nice for you to pick up Jan. I look forward to Monday.

Sleep tight. I'll dream of you.

- Abbe

Email from Abbe to Jim,
October 2014

It feels odd this time, leaving you in Seattle to visit my mom. Besides missing you, I feel as if I'm floating between moments.

I woke with fuzzy eyes. Tired, with a splash of sentiment. Last night Harriet came into my bedroom and lay on the other bed. We talked about the next steps and my sense of Mom's well-being. At one point last evening I saw the resigned look on my Mom's face, a dash of fear floating in unshed tears that pooled within the lids. A deer in the headlight gaze, a deep sigh of understanding that the road held bumps and that the forest slowly had disappeared. Just a fleeting moment, and others held laughter, sighs of peace. Mom retreats from large conversations. She has no patience for discord, the news, or controversy. She craves happy endings. The gift I'd like to bestow has no wrappings, no bows tied neatly. My gift would be the guidance toward peace, a hand-held embrace of all the love she has exuded throughout time. To bundle her with my own cushion of understanding and let her drift pain-free from this universe into the next.

My fuzzy eyes leave tears on my cheeks.

Mom steals from her reserve and serves love on a silver platter.

Email from Abbe to Harriet,
October 2014

Dear Har,

I believe Mom doesn't have fear or anxiety for herself, just a sadness for leaving us all behind. She knows that one day she will sleep and not wake up. She'll avoid pain and is surrounded by love. Mom knows who she is, knows what she has done, and wants for nothing. She is full. I'm not quite as brave. I hurt inside behind my ribs and feel the loss creeping up to my Adam's apple. I only want to hold Mom's soft hand. I'd like to talk with Dad, and Bubbie and Grandpa Abe, to tell them that their favorite lady will be with them soon.

Love you,
Abbe

Email from Abbe to Jim,
October, 2014

Dear Jim,

I woke ready to be here, ready to go with this new flow.
Oh, to be able to keep the calm.
Ease the transitions from angst, reaching for breath
as the body fights the mind.
Breathing thoughts as the body wants to let go.
Holding so tight to control.
Harriet and I see Mom's struggle with bills.
Hearing gone, patience out the window.
Delicate balance assisting or taking over.
Pride, elegance, determination, indomitable spirit.

∞

I kiss Mom's forehead.
I listen, laugh, stand back.
I create calm within my heart
to flow where tears go.

Missing you,
Abbe

Black and White Spectrum
A Eulogy

My mother passed away. These words seem so final and exact, like the black and white colors that populated my mom's clothes, her house. Yet within the lines of grace and elegance and tenacity, my mother's life held the spectrum of light's reflections.

I see her long piano fingers, nails painted with a pale pink polish, cupped to receive my hand. A gesture from when I was a child, a way to communicate without words, that no misunderstanding can withstand. The human touch, love in a basket.

My mother passed away. But not her lasting influence. She once told me that she regretted not going to college, not pursuing a degree. My response came with force, "How could you think that you didn't have an education? You are studied in people, politics, finance, art, philosophy, and negotiation." Humble in pursuit of excellence, she missed seeing she was a star circling this earth.

I see her with white wine, sitting with her feet thrown over the armrest of the sofa. A counterpoint to the erect posture of societal perfection, the face she gave her public. She is the comedian, storyteller, revealer of the romantic.

My mother passed away. Yet her indomitable spirit still roots for the underdog, the happy endings. She faced life, hers and that of her loved ones, as a director wanting to control outcomes, but knew that her best position was on the sidelines acting as a coach, nudging the best out of all those she believed in. Last summer she asked repeatedly to hear how I met my Jim, the romance that followed. She relished in my fairy tale.

I see her with her financial wizardry, pencil sharpened, pages of figures, as she looked for clues to erase the bad news of my husband's cancer. She searched for a miracle, and her love and devotion to Jim and me gave me the strength to find new intimacies in caregiving. Even with her own diagnosis of cancer, she took one more trip to visit me, Jim, her grandchildren, her new great-grandchild Paige Selma Porter. My sister, her travel guide, and I relished in her celebration of generations.

My mother passed away. And in her last years, the weight of difficult times lifted. She retired from real estate, the queen of Rancho Mirage after nurturing her soul mate, our father, to his rest. Her easy smile, wit, and sense of adventure poured outward for all the world to see. New friends made at bridge games, old friends, and family benefited from her stories, wisdom, and laughter.

I see her with hair teased into a bun, pale pink lipstick to match her nails. Sparkling like the diamonds she adored. Even in her last days, she sat on the stoop with me, dressed in a black cashmere robe, waiting for my cab. She clung to my arm and said, "The only reason I'll let you leave is to return to your Jim." There is nothing final in her passing. Hidden within the black are the colors of passion, and in the white, the purity of her heart.

My mother passed away. Her spirit shines within us all.

∞

Email from Abbe to family,
November 14, 2014

I wake this morning in my mother and father's home, after all the fanfare of the funeral, the reception, and then the grandkids' evening bonding. I've picked up the remnants of their youth, too much wine, chocolate cake crumbs, empty water bottles. I stack the dishes, then carefully wash the delicate stemware. My Mom should walk out any minute and smile, saying, "What a great celebration."

In this world, one so far from my home in Sedro Woolley, I sit as I have for thirty-some years in the respite of acceptance of many lifestyles, world views. Yesterday at one of the hardest moments, my new family appeared out of nowhere, to reinforce my resolve, to keep my heart pumping with love. I am so thankful the Wiggins family came into my life. Thank you Johnny and Jan, Gracie and John for traveling the distance. Rich and Shirley for being here in spirit, for always offering support. Steve and Larry for caring about Jim's wife, and for my Jim who made this happen.

Love,
Abbe

Email from Jim to family and friends, December 2014

Hi, all,

To state simply, over this past year the process of my developing cancer is this. First recognizing something was wrong with my body, then going to the doctor who diagnosed my ailment as osteopenia. Then came the cancer diagnosis and the shock, going through treatment, and now recuperation. The majority of the recuperation is getting over the therapy. It brought me close to death twice in order to kill the cancer within me. I'm still light-headed, with some fatigue, my GI is queasy, and my back is still broken.

Abbe and I are now officially out of our temporary condo living in Seattle and back home. I am certainly not at 100 percent, or back to feeling "normal," but I do feel better than I have for this past year. Thank you, medical community.

One does not travel down the cancer path alone, although some people do, and that is a sad thing. I believe I would not be here now if not for all the support I have received. My original and local doctor, who identified the cancer and immediately got me on a protocol to eradicate the wonky myeloma genes from my body, likely was my saving grace. His expertise was and is oncology/hematology. This wonderful man had worked at the Seattle Cancer Care Alliance, had experience with Multiple Myeloma, and knew the newest therapy path to put me on. That included a regime of chemo (Velcade, Revlimid, and

Dexamethasone). Those three drugs fought the cancer and reduced my plasma cell count from 80 percent of my blood to less than 1 percent. As I lived with cancer, both the irradiation of areas of my body where the myeloma was concentrated, and the chemotherapy, reduced the pain. However, because myeloma remained in my body, and because I had a mutant P-53 gene, I was considered a high-risk case. Therefore, my doctor introduced me to the SCCA, where I spent the last 6 months undergoing a tandem transplant of my stem cells.

A strong caregiver who is present at all appointments, someone to make sure to understand the medications I was on, drive, help me eat and drink, also kept me alive. There were times when I could have been hospitalized and closer to death, especially after each transplant when I lost weight and had "chemo brain," when fatigue and the inability to think normally overpowered my psyche. I am thankful that this didn't happen.

The fortune of having a perfect match of my stem cells from a family member for the second transplant also kept me out of the hospital and will prolong my life. My reference to being in the hospital is where my body would have responded poorly to the transplants or medications, and would have brought me closer to death (fever, weight loss, kidney malfunction, vomiting, and dehydration).

The last month in Seattle allowed my body time to equilibrate with Richard's stem cells, as they slowly "took over" my immune system. I remain vulnerable to his immune system, referred to as graft versus host disease. Which is where his immune system, now mine, could attack parts of my body. If this occurs, I'd be back on a heavy dose of medication or in the hospital.

The good news is I've been one of the SCCA's better patients, which I believe is, as mentioned above, due to my doctor, Abbe, Richard, the support I have had from family and friends, and the virility of my Wiggins/Carleton bloodline.

Generally cancer is not showing up in any of my analyses. However, my M-Spike remains at 1%. The M-Spike is a concentration of a particular protein that is a part of the myeloma. That protein will slowly be filtered out of my body, and my new immune system will also demobilize it so my body can filter it out.

I will have Velcade shots twice a week for 9 months and will go back to the SCCA in September to have a series of tests to check for cancer and to have a regimen of immunizations, because the treatment rid my body of all shots since childhood. Thus I remain susceptible to diseases, so I need to be vigilant.

I am not retiring, but will be slowing down a lot from work and just puttering around the house. Abbe and I are planning a host of traveling because there are a lot of memories we'd like to create. Thanks for all your support.

- Jim

Home Again
(December 2014)

Jim and I are home again. Not the temporary guilt-laden, sneak away from the Seattle Cancer Care Alliance weekend trip, but one sanctioned by our doctors. We moved our temporary offices, bedding, food, closet of medicine, and seven months' wardrobe from our Seattle apartment back to our expansive paradise of twenty acres and a house with nooks and crannies that set the stage for living.

Our release came with a ninety-minute exit class filled with warnings. Of all the attendees, Jim was the only tandem stem cell transplant, which meant he not only had to worry about the side effects of heavy chemotherapy and radiation treatments, but also had to manage the complex nature of immune suppression drugs, the fear of graft versus host disease, and the real probability that a new type of cancer could arise from the protocols as well as a recurrence of multiple myeloma. The list of forbidden behaviors and almost certain negative consequences left us wondering about freedom and life.

I ponder where a year went. I have haunting memories of Jim's broken back, the excruciating pain for him to bend, dress, and roll over. The diagnosis three months after hunting season that gave a name to his pain. Cancer explodes with ramifications. Fed by toxins, hormones, sugar, sun, stress, genes, and the unknown, cancer infiltrates the pores of our soul. Treatments filled in the holes, as the day to day regimes tunneled our vision. We no longer looked forward. I recollect the shedding of Jim's fast-growing cells, the sloughing off of hair, skin, and his innards, the lining of his stomach and colon. Jim's eyes reflected his story as we progressed through mobilizing his own stem cells for his auto transplant, his acceptance of his brother's stem cells, and the violent assault to his system with drugs that protected and killed.

The blur of procedures lingers as a reminder of Jim's progress. Odd as it may seem, I count our blessings in our bedtime snuggles. I equate love in all its forms, from the sensual touching to the comfort of hugs and holding hands, as the boldest of indicators that life is worth the push. Freedom comes with understanding the depth of fatigue. Jim, at his worst, slept. He allowed his brain the luxury of quietude, so his body healed. But with progress comes the awakened knowledge of loss, the withered muscles, the absence of strength, and the frustration of "normalcy."

Jim wakes with a list of to dos. Water plants in the greenhouse, snip the blackberry limbs before spring, fill the birdfeeders, find new compost bins, soak beans for soup. He works in his home office on bids for new jobs, payroll, paying bills. Before he even has his breakfast, his energy passes, and the big brown chair calls out his name. He never knows what to expect, but he receives what he is given. We plan not the specifics, but the general, so that our life becomes more a concept. Exercise means doing in any form. Travel isn't just a vacation place but the studying of where to go, the history, the culture, the anticipation. This has always been our way, but the new normal takes into consideration that every action must be valued.

∞

Uncertainty hides behind the fatigue, but our presence in each day gives rise to our future.

I pattern my days with Jim's. We've achieved a rhythm not guided by a calendar. Although I still set up Jim's weekly medicine regime and accompany him to our local physician for chemo maintenance treatment every other week, my role has changed. I, too, must find a new normal. I do less for Jim, and more with Jim. My future rests with deeper discovery. I also have a to-do list, but I have yet to write down new goals. I seek what I have always sought, intimacy with grace, peppered with passion and understanding. Now I want to leave a legacy of process.

Cancer doesn't belong in anyone's home or future. Death, sadness, and loss have filled this year. Yet we are home, freer than ever to enjoy the irregularities of nature, to plant our garden, to plan a trip, to share meals with family, to write short stories, to sleep deeply and snuggle. With all that is forbidden, we take joy in life. Who knew that survival included so much love?

Home again, within the unknown, we take comfort.

Utterances

I'd like to tie this past year into a tight bundle, toss the journey through cancer into the garbage and forget. But Jim's cancer doesn't disappear. It's wrapped as a gift of survival, and daily he unravels the fragile layers. Life at home is not the same as before.

Jim runs errands, shopping for dinner: lamb, shrimp, and fresh vegetables. We play tug of war over who will bring in the wood for the woodstove. I relinquish my morning ritual from this past winter, returning it to the man of the house.

Jim stores his energy. His blue eyes, bright and mischievous, shine with plans for a walk along the dike to spot great blue herons and bald eagles. Plans change midstream, sometimes just after breakfast. He takes the newspaper to read, a pause to recoup from the exertion of cooking and eating. Soon his eyes close and his head nods. He dreams the possible.

Stress seeps through cracks of bravery, emotions leak. Jim was so strong throughout all the treatment: the chemo, the pokes and prods of bone marrow biopsies, the mobilization of his stem cells, the two stem cell transplants. Now he just has to thrive. He's no longer at the peak of cancer, but his job is to be cautious. Caution drains our adrenaline rush for a cure—worn as an armor for over a year, our potent shield of protection. Now Jim and I become human again, and neither of us trusts wild abandonment. We can't quite relax. Fatigue holds us captive. We are the guards against graft versus host disease. We are the sentinels of quiet listening. Tears slide down a now clean-shaven face. They come after watching a sappy movie, or when the words "died after a courageous battle with cancer" are heard on the radio.

After a year of a scraggly beard, Jim shaves daily, a reward for platelet blood levels that remove the risk of excessive bleeding. Progress taunts us with vigilance. We monitor blood pressure and blood tests as indicators of his internal health. Jim's questions to the doctor diminish, not because he knows everything. He holds back the big question, the one that goes back to statistics. Has the cancer disappeared? Silence replaces adrenaline. Knowledge binds us to facts, when we need dreams.

When the doctor smiles with good news, we hold our breaths. "Jim, you are CR." CR translates to complete remission. Isn't this what every cancer patient wants to hear? But I know it is a trap, one that brings us back to odds. The followup to this news is the question, "What does that mean in terms of prognosis, life expectancy?" Silence, then the quote, "Sixty percent of patients stay in complete remission for up to five years." I think of the forty percent who don't. I know that there are no statistics past five years. NO ONE KNOWS.

The smile vanishes from the doctor's face. He warns Jim of his failing kidneys. That his blood draws show an abundance of creatinine. His body isn't flushing out his medications. If there isn't an improvement with the next blood draw in a week, Jim needs to go back to a kidney specialist for a biopsy. He is told not to worry, just drink three liters of water each day, and we'll see.

Jim vows to be accountable. He has his jug to pour out the glasses of water. He is faithful, even adding an extra glass of water to compensate for his glass of wine.

Jim and I celebrate time. The new and old. *Newold*, the place where statistics can't be measured, where we take time for a soak in our jetted tub. This is the grand pause marking our first submersion in water, without doctors' warnings, since October 2013. Yesterday Jim walked to the railroad tracks, an additional half mile past our mailbox. The greenhouse attached to our home thrives. All their dead leaves gone, watered and rotated, the plants appreciate Jim's attention. Why look at the big picture when the small ones are so beautiful? We can't wait for a diagnosis on our life. Both prognosis and diagnosis limit our view. I will not fill the black hole of the unknown with judgments.

Jim's hair has changed. I look at his new hairdo, the gray-white wisps and spring coils that wave into rippled edges at the back of his head. His crown, a high rise of rule-less curls above his forehead, creates the mad scientist aura. His brother thinks he looks like his mother. I see a baby chick with fuzz. I wait, not for utterance of cures, but for the fuzz to shed and sprout colorful feathers, so my Jim can soar.

∞

Epilogue

"Period"

Whenever Jim is emphatic about a thought, or concept, he adds at the end of a conversation the word *period*. You can't dispute thoughts because they now are facts. The dot at the end of the sentence closes the door. End of Story.

Cancer won't allow him this luxury. No matter how long it has been, whether he heals or regains strength, a visit to the doctor's office removes the certainty. Jim is in a trial maintenance program, which adds a layer of both risk and caution. The trial protocols call for nine months of chemotherapy. In Jim's case it is Velcade, part of one of the original cocktails, to eliminate the cancerous myeloma cells. Doctors have a theory that just in case the two stem cell transplants weren't enough, this will give Jim better odds.

Odds open the door to risk, and risk opens the door to doubt and worry. What if Jim's brother's stem cells haven't engrafted, contrary to the desired result? What if the absence of graft versus host disease, Richard's immune system, fighting Jim's immune system, reveals that Jim's system won't give in to the change? Jim, the little brother, would finally win over his oldest brother. To win means loss. The benefit of the new immune system would have been wiped out without any signs of discomfort. The battle to control the myeloma would make it appear that all is well. The extra doses of Velcade could have helped Jim seem normal and hindered the process. Would it be better that their systems continued the battle for a longer time?

Yesterday marked six months since the allogeneic stem cell transplant. Instead of a celebration, the doctor performed another bone biopsy. As he lay on the operating gurney, Jim asked a question that gets to the core confusion. What are they monitoring, the cancer, or him? Is there a difference? Can you monitor absence?

I'm not fazed by the marrow aspiration, the dark vial of stem cells. I watch as a piece of bone marrow slides out like a red inchworm. I ask about chimerism, as if the term were part of my everyday vocabulary. They will test for the percentage of brotherly takeover and see if Jim's blood type is now that of Richard's. We wait for results.

I believe that the trial protocols layer a sense of security above all the science and doubts. The doctors observe the changes in Jim. They are not in control of cancer. Cancer isn't the story. There will never be a period, there will never be an end to Jim's story. He lives forever. The next chapter continues...

∞

Caregiver's Tips

I wish I had the answer to questions not yet formed. Everyone's journey through cancer is unique. Different cancers, different bodies, different lifestyles, different support systems, and different wills merge to create a healing atmosphere. Jim, as the patient, credits me with a strength I don't have. I credit him with a spirit of hope mixed with the fatalism of facts. Somehow we forged a unit of deeper love that carried us forward. The following tips reflect my own insights to questions I had along the way.

Fear

When Jim's diagnosis came, I worried about driving in Seattle. I hate to drive and focused on my known fear rather than on the big issue of dying. This served me well as I learned to drive to and from the SCCA, and I communicated what I couldn't do to the staff. They gave me vouchers for late-night taxi trips to the hospital or doctor's visits that had me travel out of my comfort zone. We forged a dialogue of openness. When the time came for me to deal with the harder fears, I found that I no longer fainted at the sight of blood, that I could withstand the rigors of watching difficult procedures. My hands were steady as my heart.

I still hate driving. Jim is back at the wheel.

Finances

Keep life simple. Consolidate all your bills. Refinance to free up cash flow. Have all your regular bills paid automatically so you don't have to worry about missing payments. Let the banks know your situation.

If you run a business or work outside of the home, find a way to work remotely. I bought new laptops and saved everything to the "cloud." Each day I woke up early, and by the time Jim had his appointments, I had balanced my restaurant's books, made orders, posted payroll. I found that on my return to home, I could take more time off.

Health Insurance

Jim and I pay our own insurance. With the new Affordable Care Act, we found out that there isn't a cap on cost for Jim's treatments. Premiums and the deductibles were our only expenses. This gave us a maximum out-of-pocket amount and took the uncertainty out of the future. We made sure that every procedure requested for Jim fell under "covered" expenses and had paperwork that validated approval. Jim had to choose between two different experimental trials. One had coverage and the other, while promising, was too new for our plan to cover. This made our decision easier. We didn't second guess ourselves. Coordinate with the doctors and hospitals beforehand.

Honesty

A second pair of eyes to watch, another ear to listen, keeps everyone on course. When Jim was first diagnosed, his ears refused to listen to time frames and procedures. He could take in the immediate facts, but the long-term prognosis escaped him. Often I'd stare down at my notes and wonder if we had been in the same room. I believe his mind protected him from the fact that we'd be involved and away from home for seven months. He'd repeatedly tell everyone his version. They'd call me later for another version.

At the doctor's office, tell what you observe, not what the patient or doctor wants to hear. Refrain from making excuses, or reasons for why you think something is happening. Allow the doctors and nurses to use their knowledge unbiased by your opinions.

I noticed that most people held onto positive information and let the harder points dissolve as if they didn't exist. Only late at night, when our defenses slipped away, could we whisper truer thoughts. Each of us came to the same place with the disease, but our timing wasn't always in sync. Even the doctors doled out information that seemed contrary. How could there be so many interpretations of the same facts? For complex situations, the brain can absorb only a certain amount. Often it wasn't what you asked that mattered, it was the sigh of the newest doctor on duty that told you more. Keep optimistic, but don't confuse truth, difficult stages, with pessimism. Truth keeps you prepared.

Pain

The first question with each visit began with, How is your pain level? In the beginning, Jim would underplay the pain. Ten seemed inappropriate. The number always hovered around three to six. After many days of holding my tongue, I finally spoke up. "Please multiply Jim's answer by two, and then you will understand that Jim has a high tolerance for pain. He is not a complainer." His verbalizations of "gugh" when he bent over, or walked, or tried to get off the toilet seat, clued me in to what he refused to believe. Later during the months of treatment, Jim would be able to make comparisons to prior weeks, or pinpoint differences.

∞

The best advice for managing pain is to stay ahead of it. Jim, like many people, despises taking pills or any type of medication. He learned the hard way that pain depletes the body of energy and the ability to heal. He found a non-narcotic pill that works. Worries of addiction come when there is no pain. All prescriptions have side effects, but pain debilitates the patient.

Medical Bills

To stay on top of the medical bills, I devised a system of payables like that of any business, with packing slips and invoices. The appointment schedules became packing lists of sorts. They detailed all blood work, procedures, and doctor and nurse meetings. I filed them by month. When the insurance summary came in, I'd check off the charges by day. All of the insurance notifications state that this is not a bill. Bills come from SCCA, or other specialists. When I paid a bill, I could pull out the "packing list" or "schedule," the insurance's declaration of costs and patient's responsibility, and I'd be able to verify all charges. I posted in my notebook the date, procedure, total charges, and what I paid. (With seven months of treatment, I found two errors, which were rectified after calling our insurance and the SCCA.)

Make sure all procedures are pre-approved and are coded appropriately based on diagnosis. By the time Jim had finished his two transplants, the charges totaled close to $500,000. We paid only out-of-pocket about $7,000 dollars plus our monthly premiums. We are so thankful that we had health insurance!

Prescriptions demand two files. One for the cost, and another one for the description of the drug's purpose and side effects. I kept the description file alphabetically, so I could easily refer back. When Jim no longer needed a certain medicine, I marked an "X" on the prescription and the date when he stopped. As Jim's treatments progressed, his medicine list expanded. We now have a pill box with five slots per day. It takes me an hour each week to set up his pills. Have a cheat sheet where everything is summarized. The SCCA provided us with revised medicine lists each month. If you don't have a list, ask your clinic for an official, current guide to the reason each medicine is used. Also verify when you should take each pill, with or without food, and make sure you avoid eating grapefruit. Grapefruit messes with the effectiveness of some drugs. Note that some drugs can be affected by tomatoes, or anything from the nightshade family. Pay attention to any changes in mood or physical well-being. One of Jim's anti-rejection drugs created swollen feet that were beyond painful. Compression socks helped while they tried to adjust his dosage.

Advocacy

Many voices swirl around the caregiver and patient. I took notes, Jim listened. We both arrived at each appointment with a list of questions. The doctors, nurses, physician assistants, and other staff took time to explain, but sometimes their words made no sense. When that happened, I would repeat what I thought I understood. This approach allowed the staff to find holes in our thoughts, and forced us all to avoid accepting protocol without justification.

When the lab made their huge error with Jim's stem cell count, their explanation made no sense. All attempts at justification failed. Trust in our own voice, in our own powers of thought, kept us on target. Blame would have derailed our relationship with staff, so I focused on the outcome we all wanted. Less pain, more stem cells for the transplant, and Jim's survival. I insisted on procedural reports and offered ideas on quality control, and the ability for all voices to be taken seriously when results fell out of the norm. To be heard, voice your concerns with power, minus harshness.

Humor

Cancer isn't funny. But life is. Find reasons to laugh. Jim and I looked forward to our picks of movies each night. We avoided tragic news. We noticed everyone and smiled in the elevator. While growing up, I wanted to be a comedian, and I had a captive audience this past year. To see Jim laugh, his blue eyes smile even before his lips moved upward, egged me on. Applaud the repetition of tests, the green bag that meant a patient had to give a urine sample. Smile at pedestrians as they pass you by, because your walk resembles a tortoise with glue on its feet. Hold hands.

Questions I Still Ponder

What do you mean by Cocoon of Cancer?
The moment Jim and I entered into the world of cancer, I felt that we had left behind our normal life. A cocoon encases and protects. Jim has two tattoos, one on each arm. One is a butterfly, and one is a frog. Both go through a metamorphosis. With cancer the change is internal, and there is no guarantee that you will emerge. The world outside matters less. Jim and I view life differently from before. We saw others with cancer and connected on an emotional level. Bonds fortified and nurtured us. Even now with Jim in remission, there is a separation from the old way of living. The cocoon still holds us. We may look the same, but inside we are more aware: we care more, give more.

Why did you write this book?
I didn't mean to write anything for the public. My essays and poems were part of how I began my days. I'd get up early, before Jim woke, to find my center, to connect all my emotions. I wrote so that I could be strong for Jim. He wrote to understand scientifically the cancer and the protocols. Somehow our words made a difference to our friends and gave them an inside view of cancer. I found that the staff and doctors valued the essays. They don't often get to hear the thoughts of the patient and caregiver. The essays made us all more human and provoked questions and answers that no one anticipated.

Is this your first involvement with cancer?
Just before Jim was diagnosed, I had started writing my third novel in which the main character's twin sister had died of bone cancer. Fiction became reality

when Jim called me to tell me his fractured back wasn't because of osteoporosis and that he had an advanced stage of Multiple Myeloma. During his year of treatment, my mother was diagnosed with stage four pancreatic cancer. In breaks between caring for Jim, I'd fly down to be with my mother. Ten days with Jim, five days with my mother. She passed after only three months. I was blessed to be able to hold her hand as she left this world.

Did you ever get angry?
Of course I did. But I had only a finite amount of energy. I decided early on not to waste my time on anger. I never got angry at the cancer, or at Jim. Because Jim and I are newlyweds, married six years this spring, friends and family would ask if I felt cheated. The thought never entered my mind. My life with Jim has always been intimate. I felt honored to share the closeness, the fears, and the hard times. Whatever walls we had dissolved, and we found pleasures in just being able to eat together.

Is this a book about death?
The idea of death becomes a reality with the diagnosis of cancer. Cocoon of Cancer is about intimacy. It is about living. Neither Jim nor I changed what we enjoyed. We talked about death, but each day we made a choice. We chose to laugh more. During the procedures, the chemo, the radiation, the stem cell transplants, we didn't plan for the future. Those days, we learned. We participated in his healing. This may seem odd, but death became our friend. Jim told me the other day he now has to rethink death. I smiled. He knows life.

How did you deal with fear?
One of the caregiver tips I give in the book is about dealing with fear. For some reason I focused on my fear

∞

of driving in Seattle. I hate driving in cities or at night. I mastered the route to and from Seattle Cancer Care Alliance and voiced my fears to the staff. They supplied me with cab vouchers for times we had to travel to areas outside my comfort zone. By the time Jim had his bone biopsies, his daily blood draws, and all other procedures, I had no fear. I sat in on everything and was able to give him strength I didn't know I had.

Do you ever feel alone?
Sometimes. But Jim's journey brought out the best in all of our family and friends. By allowing others into our cocoon, we gained. They all participated in Jim's healing, and we grew closer.

Now that Jim is in remission, what is next?
We will ignore the statistics. We will continue to live our life. We will pay attention. We are still in the cocoon.

How have you been Jim's advocate?
I asked questions. I listened and watched Jim. I made sure that all protocols were followed. I volunteered to be on a review committee when there was an error in the labs. I worked on finding solutions. I respected the staff and Jim.

What would you say to those newly diagnosed with cancer?
I would offer my hand with warmth. I would let them know that the process, while difficult, is doable. That the bond begins with each of them. That they have entered into a select group of people who have values not yet tapped. Their journey will teach unsolicited lessons with invaluable results.

Questions for Readers to Ponder

What defines you? Think about what pleases you, how you want to be remembered. Then see if you can act on this now.

Do you see the doctor annually? More importantly do you know what your norm is? Blood tests are indicators and the red and white blood cells have specific jobs. Check to see any changes overtime.

Are you financial matters in order? Do you have a will? Do you have a health directive? Who will be your executor?

Think about your friends and family. Are you in a position to help them if someone gets ill?

What is your biggest fear? What actions can you do to relieve this fear?

Stress contributes to overall health. What are your stressors? What daily rituals can create a calming effect --- music, yoga, swimming ,running, writing, etc., so that you stay healthy or can endure the added stress of an ill person in your care.

This book talks about cancer, the patient, and caregiving. There are many other illness that disrupt our lives. For those readers sandwiched in between raising a family and also caring for parents the stress financially and mentally can be profound. Begin a dialogue with family members on various care situations and how they best work with your particular living situation.

Is everyone in your household covered by healthcare? With the Alternate Health Care mandate, all children, young adults, and those not at Medicare age, can find basic coverage. Prevention care not only saves lives, but the costs of a disease, major illness, or cancer is unaffordable without this safety net.

My biggest surprise when Jim was diagnosed with cancer was how quickly we had to act. Our work situation lent itself to our working off-site. Explore options with your employer. Offer to job share, work from home, or take a leave of absence.

Do you have enough in savings to pay bills for six months to a year?

Regrets eat away at one's happiness. What do you need to reconcile within yourself or with others? If you can't fix a situation, what alternatives can you manifest to create peace within?

Explore the idea of losses—people, abilities, freedom. Then explore ways to open and receive the unexpected.

About The Author

Abbe Rolnick grew up in the suburbs of Baltimore, Maryland. Her first major cultural jolt occurred at age 15 when her family moved to Miami Beach, Florida, where history came alive with her exposure to the Cuban culture and inspired her to write about her observations. At Boston University she met her first husband, a native of Puerto Rico. Her first novel, **RIVER OF ANGELS**, stems from her experiences while living in Puerto Rico and owning an independent bookstore. Later, back Stateside, she was one of the first employees at now-famous Village Books in Bellingham, WA. She now owns a healthy foods cafe.

COLOR OF LIES, her second novel, brings the reader to the Pacific Northwest where she now resides with her husband on twenty acres in Skagit Valley, Washington. Here she blends stories from island life with characters in Skagit Valley.

Her short stories and travel pieces have appeared in several magazines. "Swing Doors" won honorary mention in a *Writer's Digest* contest. Her next novel, **FOUNDING STONES**, will be the third in the series, continuing the stories of characters from the two previous novels, introducing new themes that connect Skagit Valley to the larger world.

Her recent experiences with her husband's journey through multiple myeloma inspired **COCOON OF CANCER: AN INVITATION TO LOVE DEEPLY.**

∞

CPSIA information can be obtained
at www.ICGtesting.com
Printed in the USA
FSOW01n1415130116
15490FS